STORIES OF AMAZING HEALTH TRANSF...
TRAINERS, ATHLETES ANL ... ...

TOTAL
HEALTH
FOR
EXTRAORDINARY
LIVING

LAWRENCE TUAZON
KERRY B. FISHER

WITH 28 HEALTH COACHES, TRAINERS, ELITE ATHLETES,
PEAK PERFORMERS AND WEEKEND WARRIORS

Library of Congress Cataloging-in-Publication Data
Names: Lawrence, Tuazon; Fisher, Kerry, Authors
Title: *TOTAL HEALTH FOR EXTRAORDINARY LIVING: STORIES OF AMAZING HEALTH TRANSFORMATION FROM ELITE COACHES, TRAINERS, ATHLETES AND PEAK PERFORMERS*

LCCN 2022920513

ISBN 978-1-958165-10-2 (Softcover)
ISBN 978-1-958165-09-6 (Hardcover)
ISBN 978-1-958165-11-9 (eBook)

Nonfiction, Mind, Body & Spirit, Health, Self Help

Interior Design by FormattedBooks.com

CONTENTS

CONTRIBUTING AUTHORS

The authors who contributed to this book are health coaches, trainers, elite athletes, peak performers and weekend warriors. They are on a mission to spread knowledge about holistic health and wellness to the world. These changemakers and thought leaders are part of a new wave of coaches and professionals who are changing the paradigm of health. They seek to become the very best versions of themselves and to live their most extraordinary lives so that they can teach others to do the same.

Nadia Blackstock	Claudia Valentinuzzi Núñez
Caitlyn Brightmon	Karla Ornelas
Bruno Dos Anjos	Sonal Ladwa Patel
Aaron Elsner	Nolan Pillay
Stephanie Escorial	David Priego
Freeman Fung	Andre Roggy
Lucy Hehir	Priti Shah
Kanika Jain	Irina Shehovsov
Ashutosh Khemka	Karen Stanton
Thierry Leblanc	Kimberly Stumne
Kunihiro Matsuo	Chanthy Thong
Alexandra Merlo	Nancy Yang Timmins
Patrick Morrison	Aviram Trachtenberg
Irma Nejstgaard	Amrys Wang

Dedicated to Ronan Diego de Oliveira and Lorenzo Delano

The authors in this book met through two
incredible health coaching certifications.

The Holobody Certification was created by Ronan de Oliveira and the
10X Strength Training Certification was created by Lorenzo Delano.

Quite literally, this book would not exist without them.

Ronan & Lorenzo:

We appreciate you guys so much for all the amazing work you have done
to help create the greatest health coaching certifications in the world.

Your commitment and passion for your work is an inspiration to us all.

Holobody and 10X certifications have changed each
of us on a personal level as well as creating endless
opportunities for us on a professional level.

You have equipped us with the information we need to
grow into the very best health coaches we can be.

We appreciate your dedication, your enthusiasm and your love for us.

XO Kerry and Lawrence

FOREWORD

BY TOMA MOLEROV
HOLOBODY HEAD COACH

Most of us don't care about health until we have to. And rightfully so. Life is to be lived.

I always saw health related work as the necessary, the needful, the sour part of the apple that I just had to endure. Doctors appointments, tests, surgeries, I always just wanted to 'get them over with' so that I could move on with life. But by doing that I was missing out on one of the greatest joys and mysteries of life that I'm certain you'll find yourself in the middle of when reading this book.

What if health care could be something to look forward to? Something that can deepen your relationships, enhance your business, help your family, support your team and give you something truly meaningful?

The stories in this book will give you an idea of how this may look. I had the pleasure of meeting the authors of this book during our first health coaching program that we called 'Holobody' - it was a 4-month journey, where we explored 7 lifestyle habits that would turn our life around.

Some of our authors here are doctors, others are entrepreneurs, many of them are individuals like you and me who turned their life around when health had to become the focus.

Because life is to be lived, I hope you'll take your time with this book and indulge in one story after the other. It will not only give you a different way to approach health, it will give you something much deeper, more vulnerable and more meaningful. It will give you true stories of the hero's journey towards total health transformation.

Ladies & gentlemen, it's time you meet the people behind this extraordinary book. Enjoy.

In deep gratitude,
Toma Molerov

WELCOME TO TOTAL HEALTH

The first wealth is health.

~ RALPH WALDO EMERSON

Welcome and congratulations on making the decision to buy this book. You are holding in your hands a book filled with tips, tricks and techniques for creating a life filled with abundant health and wellness. The ideas in this book have changed our lives and we are confident that if you let it, this book will change your life as well. We are so excited you have decided to take this journey with us.

This book is intended to be used as a manual where you will find many ideas for improving your health, yet it is a lot more than that. In the pages of this book, you will also find the stories of health coaches, trainers, elite athletes and weekend warriors. They share the events that triggered their health transformations and the journey they took towards total health and wellness. These are the stories of people who are sharing their journeys so that they can inspire you and make you see what is possible when you decide to take full responsibility for your body, mind and spirit. It is all about telling the truth about yourself to yourself, deciding it is time to change, making a commitment to move towards your goals and then taking action each and every day towards that vision of a healthy you. Step by step, bit by bit, you will get there.

As you read each of these incredible stories, open your heart and mind and you will see that every single one of us is capable of creating abundant health and wellness. Regardless of where you are in your health journey, we are confident that these stories will show you that it is never too late to make your health a priority. It is never too late to embrace a life where robust health is attainable. You can reclaim your health and reclaim your life.

This book shows you that health is not just about the physical, it is not just about the body. Instead, a life of health can be reached only by examining the patterns of thinking that created your current level of health. By examining your patterns and the way you think about food and exercise, you will begin to understand how you think about health. This moment of honesty may just be the most important moment on your health journey.

Once you have this moment where you acknowledge how you got where you are, you can begin to rewire your brain and change your patterns. It happened for the authors in this book and it can happen for you.

Are you ready to become the very best version of yourself? Are you ready to move into a life of incredible health and wellness? Are you ready to live the active, fun life you have always wanted?

If so, your journey begins now. Let's go!

The key to realizing a dream
is to focus not on success but significance,
and then even the small steps and little victories
along your path will take on greater meaning.

~ OPRAH WINFREY

PART I
LIFESTYLE CHOICES: INNER WORLD

Think of your mindsets as your foundation. With a solid foundation, you can build something amazing and strong.

~DAVE PEROTTA

PART I: MINDSET

We begin the health journey by focusing on your mindset. Your mindset encompasses your beliefs and your thought patterns, which were created by the information that you were surrounded by as you were growing up. This means that the views of your parents, extended family, friends, teachers, neighbors, society, religion and cultural background all contributed to shaping your mindset.

So many different influences have impacted your mindset and your mindset has created the life you are currently living. Your mindset determines your health and well-being as well as your relationships, your career, your quality of life and your ability to live your best life. One of the main themes you will find running through this book is that health is not just about the physical state of your body. Health is the totality of every aspect of your body, mind and spirit.

Examining your mindset will allow you to approach your health in a way you never have before. By changing your mindset, you will find that you can not only change your habits but you can maintain this change over time. That is the key.

The simplest way to look at mindset is to look at the idea of a fixed versus a growth mindset. A person with a fixed mindset believes that the way things are now cannot be changed and that they have no control over their situation, while a person with a growth mindset believes that anything can be changed and that they are the one that needs to change it.

In the realm of health, a person with a fixed mindset will believe that their current level of health cannot be changed. This belief creates a lifestyle where the person will not take responsibility for what they eat, how active they are or how they approach health. Typically, this leads to a life where every year the person gains a little bit of weight and gets a little bit less healthy. Unfortunately, in many societies, the idea that our bodies break down as we get older is an accepted truth which serves to reinforce the downward spiral of health experienced by so many people. When society tells us that we have no ability to become any healthier than we are, we believe it.

A person with a growth mindset, on the other hand, believes that anything can be improved. They have the confidence to believe in themselves and to create the change that they want to see in their lives. These growth oriented people take full and utter responsibility for everything in their lives, including their health. When their health is not optimal, they will do what it takes to get back on track. These growth minded people often have to disregard what they see around them and what society is telling them in regards to what is and is not possible as far as health is concerned. They seek the path where they can become the person they dream of being.

So how do you move from a fixed mindset to a growth mindset? How do you effect change? The first step is the desire to take full responsibility for where you are today and the recognition that you have a fixed mindset in some areas of your health. That's the hardest step. The good news is that once you acknowledge this, change is possible. The great news is that current research shows that you can actually change your mindset and rewire your brain.

The stories in the following chapters will detail this very journey. The journey from denial to total acceptance and then from acceptance to radical responsibility for all things to do with health. When you decide to take this journey towards self responsibility, when you go from being unconscious about your health to being fully conscious and responsible for your body, mind and spirit, magic happens.

These stories will inspire you and uplift you and most of all, encourage you to go on your very own health transformation.

The whole secret of a successful life is
to find out what is one's destiny to do and then do it.

~ HENRY FORD

Rock bottom became the bedrock in which I rebuilt my health and life.

~Lawrence Tuazon

Life takes on meaning when you become motivated, set goals and charge after them in an unstoppable manner.

~Les Brown

CHAPTER 1

REDEFINE WHAT IS POSSIBLE & LIVE AN EXTRAORDINARY LIFE

by Lawrence Tuazon

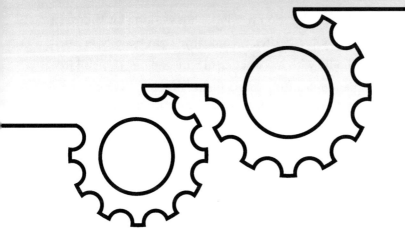

TOPIC:	Mindset
TOOL:	Empowerment Exercise
TECHNIQUE:	Ask yourself powerful questions to keep your mindset in a positive place.

I can be changed by what happens to me.
But I refuse to be reduced by it.

~MAYA ANGELOU

Difficult roads often lead to beautiful destinations and my life is a perfect example of this. Being an immigrant here in Japan for more than a decade, I'm so blessed to be where I am today. I have learned how to dream and plan my life and I have been able to make all my dreams and plans come true.

Today, I am a health and wellness coach who helps people all around the world. I have the freedom to make my own schedule and to work wherever I want because I have a location-free job. I am working for Evercoach at Mindvalley, a dream job at a dream company. I am happily married, living in a beautiful house with my wonderful wife and our two children. Even more amazing and rewarding to me is that my story is one that has inspired and created an impact on thousands of people all over the world.

I get what I plan and dream in life.

But it was not always like this.

My career was a Cinderella story. It began with my first job where I climbed from the bottom to the top of a giant retail company. I aimed for the top and excelled at everything that I did. I eventually worked my way up to the head of the department and I got plenty of positive feedback and lots of recognition. It came at a price though. I was working too much, not taking care of myself and my health was suffering. I didn't care though. Back then I had the attitude that in order for me to be successful in life, I had to sacrifice something.

I believed this formula was the way to get ahead: Success = Sacrifice.

I sacrificed my health in order to be successful. I put all of my time and effort into being number one in every job I had. Moving from department to department, I had one goal and that was to be the best. I wanted to be number one in every department that I managed and I succeeded in this. Yes, I became number one. Yes, I got the recognition and promotion that I desired. But the price was steep. I had failed at taking care of the most important thing. I had failed my body, failed my health.

The more career success I had, the more I worked. I remember that when I became part of the management team I began to work between 13 and 15 hours per day. I was eating convenience store food because I was always on the go. Back and forth I went from work to home and home to work. I was sleeping five hours per night and I did that for a full five years. Imagine that! Five hours per night of sleep for five long years.

Funny thing is, I thought that this was normal because my colleagues on the team were doing the very same thing. We were working under high pressure to achieve target sales plans and goals. We were overworked and totally stressed out. We only focused on work and forgot all about our outside responsibilities, even our families were forgotten. It was a single pointed focus on our careers, on success, on money, on moving up.

During my annual medical checkup in 2018 the doctor told me that I was overweight, close to obese. He told me that I had to come back to repeat part of the check up and to redo my blood work because of the alarming results. I remember being shocked by that.

I also remember that back then, I was exhausted most of the time. My energy level was very low and it was very hard for me to focus. I had mood swings throughout the day and I had very poor control over my emotions. After the checkup, I knew I was harming myself, I knew I had to get healthy but I simply didn't know how I could do that. I couldn't quit my job because that was the only way I had to provide for my family. For my wonderful wife and my brand new baby daughter. I had to work to give us a better life and a brighter future.

I decided to ignore my health and just keep working. I believed this was the right thing to do, but I was wrong.

You see, in addition to harming my health, I was also harming my relationship with my wife with my excessive working. We had a brand new baby to take care of but I was never home. My wife needed me to help her but I was always working overtime. By the time I came home each night I was drained and tired and all I could do was eat and go to sleep. I lived in this cycle for years. Maybe you can relate. Many of us have been on this particular hamster wheel.

Then, it all came crashing down.

It was 2018 when it happened. I was at work and there was an accident. A forklift crushed my right leg. I don't remember much but I do remember the extreme pain I was in. It was all a blur as I was rushed to the hospital. I was in and out of consciousness, everything was getting dark. I was sure that I was going to die. It was terrifying.

I lost 4 liters of blood and was unconscious for three days.

When I woke up, I was in the intensive care unit. I awakened to the sounds of my wife crying. When she saw me open my eyes she ran over and hugged me. I'll never forget her words. She said, "I'm so glad that you're awake now and still with us. Please hold on! I love you and we need you!"

I cried.

And then, I noticed my leg. It looked horrifically damaged. It was still there, but it looked truly terrible. My mind grappled with what I saw, what I knew deep in my heart.

My doctor came in and slowly, quietly, he began to speak. He told me how badly damaged my leg was. He said that my best chance of survival would be if I amputated my leg. My brain recoiled when I heard this. Amputate my leg? No! Never!

I was terrified. I did not want to lose my leg. I wouldn't lose my leg. I refused the doctor's advice. I kept my leg.

For the next six months I fought for my leg. I did anything and everything I could to recover and regain use of my leg. I underwent ten major surgeries including skin grafting and muscle transplants in my quest to keep my leg. I even moved hospitals three times in my single minded journey to save my leg. I did it all. I went above and beyond to save my leg because I simply couldn't accept the truth.

After a while, I was let out of the hospital. I wasn't functioning very well at this point. My body, mind and spirit were failing me. I was so destroyed.

When I got out of the hospital, they gave me crutches to walk. I tried to go back to my normal life, not realizing that normal life was impossible for me with my leg in the condition it was in. Every day I would try to walk around, to resume my life. I remember that I would get to a street intersection and press the button to cross. When the light turned green, I would begin to cross with my damaged leg but before I could make it across the light would begin to blink and blink. I would still be in the street, feeling vulnerable and desperate as I tried to make it across. But there I was, still in the middle of the street when the light turned red.

This happened so many times but it was only part of what was happening during that period of my life. You see, I was in a lot of pain so I started to take a lot of pain killers. As the winter cold came, my leg became even more sensitive to pain. It was getting worse and worse. My already decreased mobility was even more hampered and became less and less active. I started stress eating and gaining weight quickly. Before I knew it, I was clinically obese at 234 pounds (106 kg).

I knew something had to change so in February of 2020, in the lowest moment of my life, I decided to remove my damaged leg. The recovery from the surgery was very difficult, I felt hopeless and helpless inside, thinking that I would better be dead. I always distracted myself to escape reality by playing computer games, watching endless television series, movies and drama.

All day all I did was scroll through social media, watching other people's lives so that I could distract myself away from my own life. I could barely even look at myself. I didn't want to look at myself.

I eventually received my prosthetic leg, but learning how to use it to walk was very, very painful. It was harder than I had expected because my body weight was so heavy that I couldn't practice walking. My muscles became weaker and weaker and then began to atrophy from decreased mobility. I spent the majority of my time in my bed or a wheelchair, often not walking for months.

I couldn't go back to work and I lost the position, fame and power that I had. All of the things that I built in my career were gone. It seemed like everything that I had built was over and I didn't think life would ever get better for me. A deep heavy depression began to wave on me.

"I'm trapped in this body, I'm trapped in this life of constant pain. I have no hope inside. I don't know what to do."

I remember sitting in a wheelchair and my two year old daughter was in front of me trying to play with me. But I couldn't play. It broke my heart. I couldn't even do something simple like play actively with my baby. I couldn't even carry her on my shoulder. I couldn't walk with her hand in hand. I couldn't do anything with my daughter. This was my life.

It was this moment when I knew I had to change, This moment when I knew that I had to do anything and everything I could to regain mobility so that my daughter could have her father back again. This was the shift I needed to make. I knew something had to change in me. I knew that what I was doing wasn't working.

I had hit my rock bottom.

I was willing to let go of everything. I knew it was now or never. I had to go all in. I was ready. I wanted to give myself another chance to live so that I could reach my goals and dreams in life. I was ready.

I began doing research and learning how to live an amputee life. As I did so, I realized that my disability did not have to be a block for me to resume living my life. I knew it was part of me, but I also knew that there were many things I still did have.

I started to focus on what was working for me, which was my body and mind. I stopped cursing them and instead, I began blessing them everyday. I stopped counting what I lost. I accepted that what is gone is gone. And I asked myself "What is there left that still remains to me?"

I had my answer quickly. I had my family. I had my beautiful wife and precious daughter who supported me all throughout my long hospitalization and recovery. They were there for me when I needed them and now I wanted to be there for them. I knew they needed me. I knew they were waiting for me. So I began to heal from the inside out.

I found this miracle shift in perception, in the way I was seeing things and my situation in life. I used this exercise where I would forgive myself, empower myself and love myself. Here is the exercise:

Empowerment Exercise

I look at myself in front the mirror and call my name and ask the following questions;

Forgive Yourself
(Your Name) What do you want to let go of today?
(Your Name) What's your regret?

Empower Yourself
(Your Name) What are the things that you appreciate about yourself today?
(Your Name) How do you want to move forward and find support now?

Love Yourself
(Your Name) How can you be kind to yourself?
(Your Name) How and what do you want to celebrate today?

THE CLIMB BACK TO HEALTH

Doing this for 30 days led me to have radical acceptance of myself. I realized that it is not what happens to you that determines how successful and how happy you are going to be. Instead, it is what you do when something happens that matters.

It is not about the fall, but in the choices you make after you fall. It is the thoughts that you have about the challenge that will formulate the beliefs and attitude that you have that makes the difference. I began to realize that I was the only one who had control over my future. I was the one who determined whether I would live and thrive or shrivel up and die. It was my choice.

And I chose to live and to move towards the most vibrant version of myself I could possibly imagine.

Impossibility becomes really possible when you make up your mind. This was the mindset shift I needed to help me to bridge the gap between where I was and where I wanted to go.

I began to consume personal growth content and scoured the internet looking for information. One day, I found a platform called Mindvalley and I watched some of their free content. It spoke to me and I knew I had to join. I didn't really have the money to do this but I immediately called my wife and I told her that I wanted to enroll. At the time, we were on government financial assistance and were financially challenged by all my hospital bills. I wasn't sure how I would be able to pay. The odds were against me. And then, something amazing happened. I didn't have the money but then the money came to me just like magic. I know God and the universe supported me with my decision because I needed to change and now I was able to access the information I needed to change.

I discovered conscious health and life visioning. I started to build my mindset and heartset. I found myself stronger and better than I was before. Even better, I was finally able to play actively with my daughter. We were able to go outside and play and slowly but surely, I began to get back to my daily routine. It was like magic because I accepted and surrendered myself to the process.

All the things that I wish and plan are now happening.

I am healthy and strong. I am able to be there for my family. I have great relationships with my wife and daughter. My wife just gave birth to our second child, a baby boy. I am a conscious parent and a loving husband. My life is beautiful.

I am now working my dream job. I am giving back to the community, inspiring and transforming people's lives. I am a peak performance coach as well as a holistic health and fitness coach. I now work for the very company that I once learned from.

I regained my life.

And even though I'm now disabled, I'm able to change and transform other people's lives. My disability tells me to inspire and touch other people's lives. I am living my dreams by allowing my life to unfold as it was meant to unfold.

I have walked this journey and am here to tell you that you can walk this journey too. Wherever you are, remember, you can create a transformation in your life. Begin by doing the empowerment exercise above. It is a great starting point.

Thank you for being on this journey with me. It is my hope that we meet one day and when we do, you can tell me your story. I look forward to hearing it.

Remember, you are extraordinary and you are meant to live the life you dream of.

With love,
Lawrence

*It's not whether you get knocked down,
it's whether you get up.*

~VINCE LOMBARDI

ABOUT THE AUTHOR

Lawrence Tuazon is a health and fitness coach, a speaker and a peak performance expert. He is an amputee who has inspired thousands of people around the world with his radical health transformation.

As the founder of Total Health Coaching, Lawrence guides his clients on their journey towards peak health and fitness. Lawrence is passionate about helping his clients achieve permanent health and body transformation by encouraging them to take a holistic approach to achieve extraordinary health. His clients get results due to Lawerence's dedication to creating a tailored plan that works for them.

Lawrence is passionate about all aspects of wellness including nutrition, exercise and mindset. His vision is to create chronic health as the new normal instead of chronic disease and to bring holistic health education into the school curriculum. Lawrence believes that everybody can lead a life of extraordinary health and wellness and he has dedicated his life to this pursuit.

Contact Info:
Email: lawrencetuazon84@gmail.com
Linkedin: https://www.linkedin.com/in/lawrence-tuazon-b32725239/
Instagram: https://www.instagram.com/iamlawrencetuazon/

Shoot for the moon and if you miss you will still be among the stars.

~Les Brown

Good habits don't have to be perfect, they just have to be ... if you start and keep going, you win.

~Thierry Leblanc

CHAPTER 2
MY HERO'S JOURNEY
by Thierry Leblanc

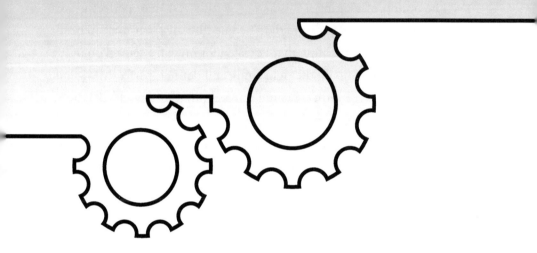

TOPIC:	Mindset: The Journey from a Fixed Mindset to a Growth Mindset
TOOL:	Body Talk
TECHNIQUE:	Tuning into your body and figuring out what your body actually needs in order to flourish.

You have been criticizing yourself for years and it hasn't worked.
Try approving of yourself and see what happens.

~ LOUISE HAY

For as long as I can remember, I had the desire and almost the need to excel and "be perfect". Being the eldest of three brothers, I always had to go through everything first, do it right to show the example and pave the way for them. I always felt the pressure to be the best, get perfect grades and to be good at everything. I wanted to do this for my brothers, but most of all, I did it to make my parents proud.

The notion of making a mistake or getting less than perfect grades became daunting. This pressure didn't come directly from my parents or my brothers, it was something that I created for myself. I moved on in life with that pressure of doing the right thing and doing it perfectly, without a misstep, because if I didn't, I could not feel proud of myself. If I didn't do it perfectly, I wouldn't feel worthy.

Along the way, many people reinforced that feeling that it is important to do things perfectly. School teachers, sports coaches and other academically gifted children were always there to let me know that if you do something, you might as well do it flawlessly. How that got engraved in my brain is: "If you can't do something perfectly, why bother? It's not worth it to spend that energy on something that is not going to be perfect." This thought was always at the forefront of my mind. I lived my life on autopilot for a while, meeting the expectations of others and trying to find myself at the same time.

I went to high school, then to university and got my bachelor's degree in engineering. After graduation, I was hired as a production supervisor for a pulp and paper plant. It was a good job, but it wasn't my calling. I obtained a lot of valuable knowledge, learned life lessons and forged my character. I found myself working hard and doing a lot of hours, but I didn't feel valued.

After a couple of years and the birth of my wonderful daughter, I transitioned to an engineering position where I learned different things but somehow, I still felt that I was on autopilot. It felt like I was not living the life that I was meant to live. Then came my second child, my wonderful son. Somehow, that is when things began to change. You see, up until that point, I had always lived with a victim mindset. I always had a good reason not to be the best version of myself. I found myself constantly making excuses. I was too busy, too tired and I didn't have enough money.

I had developed a pattern where I would start a lot of good habits and stick with them for a while but somehow, I always ended up giving them up. In fact, I would even say that I developed the habit of giving up. Maintaining good habits was hard for me because I had to follow my action plans and resolutions to perfection without any hiccups. This meant that if I started something and didn't execute it perfectly, I would lose interest and abandon the effort.

The need for perfection that I had adopted as a child made it very hard for me to stick with new habits. Whenever I was doing something, I heard that voice reminding me, "If you can't do something perfectly, why even bother?" The pressure of performing was always there, even if no one was there to put it on me. I was old enough to put it on myself. When something was hard, I would often procrastinate, find a way to forget about it and turn to a new shiny thing that seemed more interesting.

One day, one of my coworkers told me the hard truth: "You can do whatever you set your mind to. Stop using excuses. Stop giving reasons why you are not doing what you know you need to do." I don't know why but these words stuck with me. It's amazing how one sentence can change your life. I decided to examine myself and I realized that my mindset was what was holding me back. My need for perfection and fear of making a mistake was a mindset I knew I needed to change. And so it began. I started shifting my mindset slowly. I began to listen to motivational speakers and I learned the meaning of the word "accountability."

While going through the ebbs and flows of my mindset transformation, I discovered personal transformation. At first, I started with youtube masterclass videos centered on health, consciousness and a variety of topics that were at the core of the transformation I wanted to go through.

One day I heard about a health program called Holobody. It got my attention but the seminar was taking place on a weekend and with a full-time day job my weekends are mainly spent with family. I intended to try and catch as much as I could, but without any expectations. The session that I watched changed my life. In the session, the host, Ronan Diego de Oliveira discussed a concept called "body talk." Body talk is a way to get in touch with your body in order to tune into what your body really needs.

The session changed me and it changed my mindset. Listening to that session was the first time I realized that I was not cultivating a healthy relationship with my body and that I needed to change. Up until that moment, I was usually complaining about my body. I blamed the pain I had from my old college football injuries for impacting my ability to work out and get into shape. I had a lot of excuses for why I was out of shape and overweight. I had never taken responsibility for my own body or health.

After that first body talk moment, though, everything changed. I talked to my body like I would to a friend and thanked it for everything that it helped me accomplish in my life. I appreciated my body for the very first time. I also realized that the pain I felt was a cry for help and a clear message from my body letting me know I had to change. I realized that my body had taken care of me for my entire life and now I needed to start taking care of it. That realization spurred me into action.

I decided to get into shape and at the same time, I made the decision to do a Holobody Health Certification. That seminar had impacted me so strongly I had a feeling inside that I had to do it. My whole body was telling me to dive in, even if it was a huge commitment in time and money for me at the time. When the coach certification training started, I began practicing intermittent fasting (IF) and I also started my physical training using a program called 10X.

I had tried to do both of these before about a year earlier, but I had given up when I could not do it perfectly. At the time I had thought to myself that if I could not sustain this habit perfectly, every day, 'I might as well not bother at all,' so I had given up. This time around, though, it was different. I had decided that I didn't have to be perfect. With my intermittent fasting, I decided to go with a more liberal approach, to create a goal that would be achievable. My mindset went from 'Do it perfectly, for as long as you can' to 'Make it sustainable, so it lasts forever and creates a real shift in your health over time.'

My mindset went from quick temporary change to slow and steady sustainable change. To make that shift possible, I knew I needed to change the rules in my playbook. I needed to replace my usual habit of giving up after the first or second mistake and replace it with the idea that as long as I am making progress towards my goals, it really didn't matter if I skipped a day or two.

I finally understood that the only thing that truly mattered was that I keep moving forward, that I keep sticking to the plan as best as I could. I finally realized that the key to success was to implement these new habits without creating too much stress and pressure on myself. At the time I write this chapter, it's been more than a year now and I am still practicing intermittent fasting at least five days per week! I find it easy, sustainable and it is an integral part of my routine. Something that I found helpful in making it happen was to replace the routine of eating breakfast with the routine of brewing my own coffee from whole coffee beans.

Once I had the intermittent fasting in place, I turned to focus on exercise. I was using a system called 10X which was created by Lorenzo Delano. It is a system where you exercise twice per week and it fits perfectly into my life. I was on a roll! Everything was going smoothly. I was thrilled and before I knew it, I had been doing my two workouts per week for six weeks. I was proud of myself and proud of my progress.

Then, I was tested. My gym closed for renovation and then I went on vacation. There's nothing like a good roadblock to test your commitment and make you slowly but surely give up on a habit when you thought you had everything under control! I have to say that this time, these roadblocks didn't affect me as they might have in the past. That was because my mindset was different. Even though from the outside it might look as if I gave up, in my mind, I knew I would start again and make it happen.

My perspective of the situation was making all the difference in the world. This was not a failure, but a learning experience. When I would start again, I would be more equipped to face these roadblocks and keep going. I felt super empowering because I knew that I was in control of what I do and temporary roadblocks were just that, temporary. For that reason, I consider this experience a good lesson and I look forward to starting my training again!

Coming back to the coaching certification, two months in, everything was again 'under control' and I had embraced an 'unofficial' leader role inside the community of students. I was loving my role as a support person in the community and felt that I was doing something important for which I was valued. I also started to love the idea to become an ambassador for the program. Then, another vacation happened!

The coaches knew that everyone would have their vacation at some point during the training and they had let us know that it was OK to miss a week or two and to 'catch up' after coming back. As you may guess, though, my need to be perfect and ahead of the curve came crawling back into my mind. During the vacation, I felt as if I was getting more and more behind and that I was not able to fulfill my, self given, community leader role as I would have liked. The more I was having that internal dialogue, the more I became distant with the community and felt overwhelmed with the program and everything related to it. I was slipping back into the old victim mindset I thought I had conquered.

One day, during a coaching session, my coach told me: "Thierry, instead of stressing about being behind in the program, not being there for the community and distancing yourself from it, why don't you start to interact with it again to the best of your knowledge, support other students and see how it feels?" I was so scared of being unworthy to resume my leadership role within the community and to become an ambassador for the program because I was behind. I had lost sight of the fact that I was seen as valued and helpful to the community I was. After that coaching session, I started to interact with the community again.

I decided to write a message to the program manager to explain my internal struggle. He replied to me with nothing but empathy and love. He reassured me that I was and had always been a great candidate to become ambassador. His message and the interaction with the community made me feel good and valued again. I understood that from the beginning, this worry and uncertainty had always been only in my head. I continued to support the community and never looked back. Today, I am the proud ambassador of the Holobody coaching certification program.

I can think of two core insights from this experience. The first is that I am perfect and enough as I am. I bring a lot of value to people just by being myself, even though I know I can always improve. My second insight is, like Jeanette Jenkins says: "You get out what you put in. If you want more, give more."

I honestly think the biggest take away from my whole journey is inspired by my daughter listening to this song on repeat: 'Let it go.' Let go of your need to control everything. Let go of your expectations. Let go of your need for perfection, it is the mental block that is keeping you away from moving forward. When you start something that you know is going to make your life better and you keep going at a sustainable pace without ever accepting giving up as an option, you are already winning the game of life. The only way you are guaranteed to lose is if you give up. Let go of the pressure you put on yourself to meet the expectations of others. Let go of the need to always move forward and accomplish everything right now.

It is okay to breathe and sometimes take one step backward to evaluate if you really are going in the direction that you want or if you are just following what everyone else is doing. Once you've pondered that question, your vision is clear and you know what you want and it is easier to take two steps forward in the right path. You are playing the long game, or as Simon Sinek would say: 'The infinite game.' Learn to follow your intuition, trust yourself, find what works for you, focus on your strengths and make sure everything you do is in harmony with your core values.

Another concept that I heard a lot of times but had trouble integrating was: 'Trust the process.' It is so hard to trust the process when you don't see results in the short term. I found another model that is more tangible for me: 'It's all about learning to love the journey.' Instead of focusing on the results and what I would get out of it at the end, I had to find ways to enjoy the journey and see how I could make all the small steps of the journey enjoyable for me.

It's all about having the right key performance indicators.

Here are some examples:

- Instead of using my weight on the scale as a key performance indicator, I started using the way I felt and my energy level that day.
- For my nutrition goals, I started to really be more conscious about what my body was telling me. After eating processed foods with added sugars, I started noticing that I didn't feel so good in my belly, even though I didn't eat that much.
- For my workout program, I started noticing how daily tasks that were hard for me before became easier to perform.
- To monitor my stress level, I pay attention to my overall patience and reaction to unforeseen situations.
- For my energy level goal, I started paying more attention to all the different factors that were influencing my energy throughout the day like the time I went to bed and woke up, the food I ate, the supplements I was taking and my physical activity. Even the amount of sun and connection to earth and nature were having an impact on my energy level throughout the day.

Today, I am still working daily on my mindset. I am working on being audacious and leaving my comfort zone to reach new heights! We are all on a hero's journey. Even when it feels like the world is against us, the pain is just temporary and it is a challenge to make us grow, learn something new and evolve. We are never put in front of a challenge that we can't overcome!

What I think sums it all is: 'It's all about the mindset!'

Everything begins from the mind, including change.
So, if you want to alter your life, you have
to start with your mindset.

~ A L E X I   W E A V E R

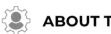

ABOUT THE AUTHOR

Thierry loves self-improvement. He is curious and passionate about everything related to health. He started his health transformation journey in 2016, when his weight hit its highest point at 300 lbs. Since then, he has worked on his nutrition, his physical exercise and several other aspects of his health! To this day, he has lost 50 lbs and is constantly working to improve.

He completed the Holobody Coach Certification and he now lives and coaches using a holistic health approach. Being the eldest of his family, he always had a feeling of responsibility to be the perfect exemplary child and pave the way for others. He lives for being able to coach and elevate anyone willing to listen and put in the work.

One of his goals is to bring his health and coaching knowledge to businesses to empower employees to be healthier and happier!

Contact Information:
Email: leblanc.thierry@hotmail.com
Linkedin: https://www.linkedin.com/in/thierry-leblanc-ing-16492017/

**If you want to go fast, go alone,
if you want to go far, go together.**

~African Proverb

CHAPTER 3
THE LIGHT BULB
by Lucy Hehir

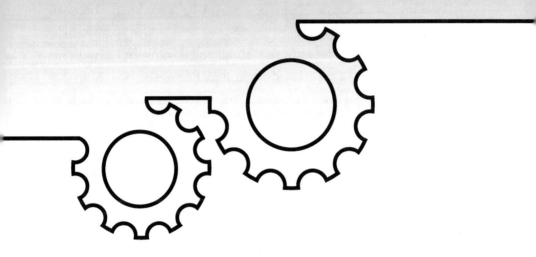

TOPIC:	Mindset: Getting Clear
TOOL:	Gaining Clarity by Allowing the Light Bulb Moments to Illuminate the Path.
TECHNIQUE:	Go on a journey of self discovery by being honest about where you are now. Reach out to friends, family members and professionals for support and encouragement.

To keep the body in good health is a duty
Otherwise we shall not be able to keep
the mind strong and clear.

~ BUDDHA

Many years ago, I was inspired by something an energy practitioner I worked with told me. She compared people's energies to lightbulbs: If you are with like-minded people, your light shines brightly and you thrive and grow from their company. On the other hand, if you were with people whose energy was not as radiant, you didn't have the same takeaway, or in many cases, you dimmed your light to fit in with them.

Looking back at my life, I can see when my light was bright and when it was not so bright.

Let me take you back to my early childhood days, when life was simple and carefree. I took for granted the healthy lifestyle of a diet of freshly grown vegetables and grass-fed meat. This was the way of life, with an abundance of clean country air on my family farm in west Cork, Ireland.

There were no organized exercise classes, no healthy eating courses as our farm chores, fun games with my seven siblings and fresh produce contributed to our beautiful, healthy lifestyle.

We rarely got sick and Granny was the go-to person when we did. She continuously reminded us, "your health is your wealth" She instilled the old healing methods. For example, a hot water bottle against our ear was used if we had an earache, bread soda in water for an upset tummy or an onion boiled in milk, vinegar in water for the anticipation of a cold and gargling with salt and water for a sore throat to name a few. We only reached out for help from a traditional doctor after exhausting all granny's home protocols.

Despite this lifestyle, I found a friend. Sugar! I just loved sugar and my favorite day was Sunday because that was the day we went to church. After church I was allowed to go to the store and buy lots of chocolate. Back then, we were not aware that consuming too much sugar could lead to severe health issues. Sugar was a treat and I ate it whenever I could.

It would astonish my family and friends how much food full of sugar I could finish in one sitting. Eating an entire packet of chocolate digestive biscuits in one sitting was the norm for me and I would still eat all my other meals. My sweet tooth continued to grow as I grew older, along with many other bad eating habits I had picked up along the way.

Before long, I was in denial about where my health was headed. I was turning fifty and honestly, I wasn't at all concerned about my health. I thought I was in decent shape "for my age." I wasn't in peak shape but after all, I was a busy working mother of two children, involved in many volunteer positions and I believed I should put everybody else's health before mine. I ate whatever I wanted when I wanted.

I slowly began having health issues and, at first, I took them as a part of getting older, as it seemed to be an accepted part of the American lifestyle. We age and our body declines. We accept this as a normal part of aging, so I was not at all worried. I could see others who were far unhealthier than I was and that somehow made me feel better.

My denial came to a screeching halt when I had a lightbulb moment at a family's celebratory anniversary dinner at a high-end restaurant. It was Christmas of 2019 when my hubby and I celebrated our 26th wedding anniversary with our son and daughter at a five-star restaurant. As I studied the menu with its delicious choices, I enthusiastically named aloud a few dishes of interest. My 15-year-old son, ever the insightful little man, said, "Mom, if you order those, it will hurt your tummy."

Wow! Out of the mouths of babes.

I was surprised and troubled to discover that I must have been complaining more than I realized —that my 15-year-old son was so in tune with the relationship between what I ate, usually gluten and sugar being the biggest culprits and how it made me feel.

Wow! Was I in denial?

How much was I complaining to my family and had they just accepted my grumblings over the years? It takes moments like these to wake up—a few simple words uttered by my son, yet so powerful to bring me to my senses. What I realized was that my sugar addiction had been contributing to inflammation and the changes I had noticed in my body as I got older.

Those words from my son started me on a mission to create a healthier lifestyle for our family. I decided to start with working on my own health. I visited my doctor, who diagnosed me with irritable bowel syndrome (IBS).

He wanted to start me on medication for IBS but having an alternative mindset, one that my granny had instilled in me, I distrusted the medical world and decided to seek help from a holistic practitioner. I didn't want to be that person who accepted taking medication for the rest of their lives without exploring other healing modalities. So I decided to seek alternative health practices- life changing practices that helped me open a healthy lifestyle I appreciate today.

The first thing I did was to get help from a holistic practitioner, Moirar. She was a challenging straight shooter, precisely what I needed to whip me into shape. At our first meeting, she explained that if I was to work with her on my health and transformational journey, I needed lots of patience and total commitment. She explained that it was like running a marathon, not a sprint, as it simply took time.

Working with Moirar, I slowly learned how my behavior had contributed to my condition. I took responsibility for my habits and my lifestyle. I realized that although it was commonly accepted in today's world, in reality, it is just a lifestyle. A lifestyle that left me feeling tired, bloated, sleep challenged. One where inflammation was an everyday occurrence and where I had accepted having gastrointestinal issues all the time. I had accepted this lifestyle, but the good news was I had it in my power to change my habits. To embrace a healthier lifestyle, one like I had as a child. A healthy lifestyle of fresh air, food from the farm, a great social environment and the natural healing methods that my granny instilled in us.

The relationship with Moirar added much light to my life. Her experience in structural techniques started me on a road where I would continue learning about my body and health, building rewarding relationships along the way and defining my true purpose. She opened my mind to different perspectives I hadn't considered previously.

We started by going deep. She had me answer the question, "Where does Lucy want to see herself, mainly healthwise, in 10-20-30 years from now?" I knew I wanted to be hiking and dancing at 80. Once I had that revelation, I knew I had to change in order to make that vision a reality. So we got to work.

My education began. I learned the importance of a strong immune system and how it was instrumental in fighting off viruses. The more I learned, the more I wanted to learn. I admit, it wasn't easy, at times patience was a challenge. Those tough moments made me understand why people opted for the magic pharmaceutical pill for a quick fix. But I didn't want that. I wanted to use natural methods as much as possible and turn to medical interventions only if I couldn't heal myself through diet, exercise and a mindset shift.

I knew it would serve me well if I kept on track, building a solid foundation. So I persisted. I changed my eating habits but, most notably, my mindset. This mindset shift was a significant shift, especially once I realized that this was not just a temporary way of eating. I remember having a moment where I thought, "What do you mean I can't return to how I was eating once I repair the damage to my gut biome? Seriously?" But then as time passed, my mindset changed, I wanted to embrace this new healthy lifestyle for the rest of my life.

Once I started seeing the benefits of my health journey, that light tummy feeling brought me back to my childhood days. I knew this natural route was for me and granny would be so proud. I was on the path to nourishing my mind, body and soul, taking all the natural vitamins and minerals and feeling fabulous. I had accepted my past lifestyle, not knowing it was detrimental to my health. Those few words my son uttered awakened my return to the alternative world for myself. I had always relied on my long-distance homeopath for my children's health, yearly flu remedies, fevers, asthma and even pneumonia, but somehow neglected to work on my own.

I was making great strides, a marathon for sure and after about a year, I decided to dive deeply into personal growth. I joined many programs and learned a lot, but one of the best platforms I found was Mindvalley. I had heard about it and as luck would have it, an invitation to join arrived in my inbox a few days later. Weird how that happens, as if someone was listening to my inner thoughts. The programs I signed up for focused on overall extraordinary holistic body wellness and they were great. Once I joined, I realized this educational platform was just what I needed.

My journey has been a long one. Mostly, it has been a journey of self-discovery of the inner me. I did it for my mind, body and soul. I was transforming rapidly and I learned to simply be open to listening and learning and taking what worked and resonated for me. I was not disappointed as I continued my marathon to health.

I learned to be more conscious of my total well-being, taking me back to basics. I added structure to my day, creating morning and evening routines. My morning routine is to rise early, drink a glass of water with salt and meditate, which helps me to be more peaceful, in tune with my life and less judgmental. Then a few words of body talk with myself. Initially, this was a bit weird, but eventually, it became easier. From these body conversations, I became aware of how badly I was treating my body.

My nighttime routine is to finish eating three hours before I go to bed (no electronics allowed). I also think about my day and the one thing I was most grateful for that day. These are still in practice and can be challenging at times, but once I'm in the zone of practice, I feel so good. I truly treasured learning about my subconscious mind and how to reprogram the patterns and habits that often sabotaged my self-image.

Learning about the root causes of inflammation, which I had plenty of, was life-changing. Inflammation can lead to many other diseases, such as heart disease, arthritis, obesity and diabetes. Educating myself on my health only validated what I needed to continue to do.

I learned the importance of strength training and muscle-building for longevity. I was never one for intense exercise, so I was delighted to discover a routine called 10X that consists of strength training with exercises such as Squats, Push-ups and Pull-ups. The mind-muscle connection came with practice and is another terrific benefit of the program. This structured strength resistance training helped me develop strength and improve my muscle mass and posture. And it only took 15 minutes, twice a week.

It is true when they say our health is connected to our human connections, which couldn't be more accurate in my case. I was initially reluctant and intimidated to join an online platform like Mindvalley with people from all over the world. But the straight shooter, Moirar, encouraged me, so I thought it best not to face her wrath. These connections with other people inspired and encouraged me to continue my health journey.

I formed lasting relationships with people from different parts of the world with diverse backgrounds. This tribe welcomed, motivated and accepted me and I never felt intimidated. As I became stronger and more confident, I learned from each one, especially the young man who said, "You need to be the product of your product." What a powerful statement; I think of it often and it inspires me in so many ways.

The experience of finding a tribe of like minded people sparked a memory from the past that I would like to share with you. I fondly remember a disco I organized, one of my most rewarding achievements as a teenager. I saw the need for a community gathering space for teens to have a place to let loose and dance and so my accomplishment was recognizing the need and then following through to make it happen.

I was so pleased with the night's success. I realize now that it wasn't because of the high number of attendees but rather the camaraderie and the look of pure happiness radiating from every participant. We bopped, twisted and twirled as the DJ blasted the sounds of Abba, Blondie and Rod Stewart. We looked splendid in our Sunday best and grinned from ear to ear as we got physical with Olivia Newton-John. This healthy feel-good environment of people connecting and dancing was pure joy and healing at its best. I believe one of my most rewarding achievements as a teenager, who grew up in the rural countryside of Ireland, took place when I was about 15 years old.

A friend and I took on the council of my Irish local traditional town when we chose to organize a disco event. Although it was only a night of dancing and fun, back then in our local community, it was unheard of for individuals outside the scope of the council, especially a local farmer's teenage daughter, to organize such an event. The local council made organizing as tricky as possible, imposing restrictions, obstacles and hoops to jump through.

Nevertheless, with the support of my friend, I prevailed and met all the obstacles. A sense of accomplishment, proving that even a 15-year-old could achieve a challenge, shining her bulb brightly when following her inner light. The night turned out to be a delightful success. The energy was ecstatic and the dancing electrifying. I realize now that it wasn't the event's success that brought me joy, but it was the look of pure happiness radiating from every participant.

Forty years later, I often wonder why I didn't continue to do more of these events. It was a one-hit-wonder. Maybe it was too confrontational to deal with the powers that be or too scary to venture outside my comfort zone. Unfortunately, I listened to my doubting inner voice, dimmed my light bulb and retreated into the safety zone of my comfortable and carefree happy farm life.

But that fateful night at the disco allowed me to see that there was more to life. And yet, it would be 40 more years that I struggled to find the meaning of that spark in my life. I knew I was put on this earth for a purpose, but I never could quite find the courage and desire to meet the challenge.

There were many light bulb moments within these forty years but, after each one, I would return into my safety comfort zone. Not really knowing why I kept doing this was frustrating. As I reflect upon this, I now understand that you are only able to truly take your health and your life into your hands when you take full responsibility and you are truly ready to create extraordinary health and well-being. This helps me to keep moving forward.

Continuing on the road to self-discovery, I joined a food freedom program recommended by one of my new friends. As one of our great philosophers, Hippocrates said, "Let food be thy medicine and medicine be thy food;" again, something that my granny lived by. But as society evolves and our lives get busy, food becomes less of a priority and we opt for convenient processed food with little thought about what it is doing to our beautiful bodies. Although it is widely known to transform our body, 85% or more is food-related and the rest is exercise.

The instructor of this optimal nutrition program that resets your relationship with food started by saying, "You are not to blame; this is not your fault." He continued to explain that we are taught the way to eat in childhood and then we never challenge those thoughts. This helped me to find a new view and helped me to somehow feel less guilty with his powerful opening statement.

This program has many different approaches than other food programs I have tried. Most notably, adding in a nutritiously green shake every morning for a few weeks before any food removals were to occur, how clever. Then when we were instructed to eliminate such things as sugar, gluten, alcohol, etc. from our diet, my body was so nutritiously happy that I did not have a lot of cravings. In addition, I learned more about recognizing and controlling my emotional eating habits, one of the six hungers. This was revolutionary for me and addressed my sugar addiction and GI issues if I stuck with it.

What we put in our gut affects our mind and what we put in our minds affects our gut. So, my mindful eating led to a very happy, light tummy and opened the door to greater mental clarity. Good health is the foundation for living. So, having a happy relationship with my body and being more educated about health, has made me more alert and more confident. I now have a better idea of my place in this world.

I woke up!

As I continued with being more conscious and more awake during my holistic health journey, I was eager to continue exploring and as I did, learning opportunities presented themselves. The last profound part of my awakening was when I attended an essential oil mini retreat. I was curious as I knew nothing about essential oils, so I attended. What happened at that retreat jolted me.

To my surprise, the attendees were asked what emotion was troubling them at that time and they spoke freely and openly about it. To my dismay through a natural process, one that the educator guided us through, our bodies picked the oil that spoke to each individual's emotional angst. Once this was accomplished, the attendees read aloud what their respective oil meant. It took me two days to process what happened at this essential oil retreat. Talk about a light bulb moment!

Some attendees arrived with troubled, perplexed looks, some with excitement and others carrying the weight of the world on their shoulders. Reading the significant meaning of the oil that resonated with their emotion sparked many awakening insights. There were tears of relief, joy, acceptance and peace in that sacred space that night. These oils provided profound support for these participants that evening and reminded us to breathe. This experience with the essential oils was the beginning of a vast exploration of healing my soul.

I created another rewarding relationship with this insightful educator as I realized my health journey also included an emotional piece.

Wow! The lightbulb moments were happening more and more frequently!

I learned that essential oils were the original medicine of the world, more natural and better for our environment than pharmaceuticals. They were illuminating the role my emotions had in all the limiting beliefs I held throughout my life's journey. Releasing these trapped feelings and energy helped with my growth. For me, they have been a true game changer but of course, this is an area that you must decide for yourself if it is something that you would like to add to your own life.

As I reflect upon this journey I have been on, I am proud of myself. I took charge of my health by taking full and total responsibility for my lifestyle choices. I learned what I needed to know in order to live the most healthy lifestyle I could. I learned about my body and what it needed, I changed my mindset and opened up to many different natural, holistic lifestyle choices. I feel better than I ever have since childhood. I have reconnected to the most important part of myself and I have learned to take care of my health, my emotions, my mindset and that has nourished my soul.

FINAL WORDS

I am grateful to my fifteen-year-old son for starting me on this journey. It was his words that began my awakening to my evolving health transformation. It is when we can remain curious and open to all the healing modalities that we can truly heal our lives.

My journey woke me up in many ways and validated what I instinctively knew from my granny. I have such gratitude for the relationships and connections that have helped me to feel lighter, clearer than ever and the confidence to share my learnings with others. It's true what the African Proverb reminds us:

I had many light bulb moments in my life but creating a stronger connection and relationship with my body makes me feel lighter and brighter with a sense of clarity for the future. This all came about because of the relationships I have formed along the way. It has been by listening to my body, caring for it with healthy foods and exercise that I have learned that it is the simple things, like getting back to the basics I did in Ireland during my childhood, that allows us to be open to the beauty of our lives.

My health practitioner started me on a marathon of self- discovery, lighting a flame that was to get stronger each time I created a new relationship. She made me realize the most important relationship I could have is with myself and that my health was the best foundation.

There are times when my light dims, but it doesn't stay that way long because I have a network to reach out to and I soon turn back to my true path. These relationships and connections have caused my inner light to shine bright and stay that way. We all need to shine and be bright lights in this world.

I am here to tell you that if I can do it, you can too. Please reach out to me to tell me your journey of how you let your light bulb moments illuminate your life, I look forward to hearing you,

Shine bright!

With love,
Lucy

ABOUT THE AUTHOR

Lucy Hehir lives on Nantucket Island with her husband Patrick. They both moved from Ireland in the 1980's. She is very proud of the light she has used to guide her two beautiful children. Her most important accomplishment is being the light she was meant to be and she likes to shine it wherever she roams. Her heart is joyful when she brings people together to enjoy an uplifting experience.

Lucy has shared her guiding light in chairing many strategic initiatives including Nantucket LIcense Plate, President of the Nantucket Community Music Center for several years, and Founder of Bridge of Culture, Irish Rambles. However, she is most excited about her cold water plunging group which shares more than cold dips in the ocean. She loves to have fun in multitudinous ways, including traveling, walks in nature, listening to music, and sharing good food with friends, She is grateful for the many guiding lights has had in her life. She loved being part of this book project and thankful for the guiding light of Lawrence and Kerry.

Lucy loves to connect with people so feel free to reach out to her and share your light!

Contact Information:
madpaddyack@gmail.com

Breathe pure air, bask in the sun, eat good nutritious wholesome food, drink pure water and observe cleanliness; you will possess a high standard of health, vim, vigor, and vitality.

~Swami Sivananda

**The universe doesn't give you what you want.
The Universe will reflect to you WHO YOU ARE.**

~Michael Beckwith

CHAPTER 4

VISION FOR THE FUTURE

by Caitlyn Brightmon

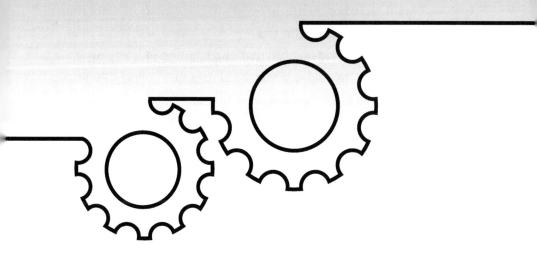

TOPIC:	Mindset
TOOL:	Visualization & Rewiring Your Brain
TECHNIQUE:	Imagine the person you want to be in the future and then merge into the emotions, the spirit of that vision. Practice this often in order to rewire your brain.

Vision without action is merely a dream.
Action without vision just passes the time.
Vision with action can change the world.

~JOEL A. BARKER

Manifest the tomorrow you want today. Visualize. Merge.

And so I practiced. Daily, I meditated and visualized where I wanted to be in one, two, three years time.

The career, the lifestyle, the body, the partner. I daydreamed in stolen minutes during the day, in seconds in between tasks, anytime and anywhere. When I prepared my meals I dreamed, as I sat crushed on public transport- train, peak hour traffic or bus, I imagined a better future awaiting me. I dreamed my biggest dreams.

I dreamt of the holiday I wished that I had, instead of worrying about the deadline I had to meet that afternoon. I dreamt of a gorgeous home, a beautiful car and a fulfilling career that I loved.

I felt guided to feel gratitude and put emotion into this vision of what I wanted. I would implore the skies, "Oh please! I want this life for myself!!" I would plead to the universe, sometimes in desperation; a lonely voice in the void.

Then, my life fell apart.

I had just had my 59th birthday. I had been in a relationship for twelve years, living with my partner for ten years at this point and I thought we were settling into the "comfortable" era of our relationship. Our partnership was passionate, loving, warm and funny. We had the house, the cars; our kids had grown, with our daughters living with us. We had our four (FUR) kids which encompassed four dingoes, an old fluffy handbag dog and a cat. My partner had his interests. Very much (apart from the dingoes) the epitome of residents currently living in Southwest Sydney, Australia.

And then, suddenly, the relationship was over. Finished. I couldn't understand it.

Why did this happen? Why? If I'm doing what the experts say, using visualization to manifest my dream life, why has it fallen apart? These were the questions I was asking myself, in April 2020.

It was a beautiful autumn day and although I wasn't consciously aware of the warmth of the sun bathing me, I felt it at some level. I was sitting on the park bench sobbing my heart out. I had come out here so no one would see me and I could let the emotion out. Trying to be a big girl.

Trying not to sink into despair. Everything I had created was crashing down around me.

Before I knew it, I was moving out of the home I had come to love because it was my ex-partner's house. I found myself being forced to move myself and my daughter out and find rental accommodation that would allow the pets.

Apart from the grief, I was angry. Back to renting. It felt like I was back where I started, in the rental world where your home could be taken from you at any time: leases not renewed, houses put on the market for sale, rental price hikes. I was all too familiar with that world. I had experienced it all in the past while raising my children as a single mum. No! Not again!

I remembered a book that I often used as a go-to when I was in limbo in the past. I had also recommended it to many of my clients over the years as I coached them through tough times in their lives. It was called *The Wisdom of Florence Scovel Shinn* by Florence Scovel Shinn.. I went back home and pulled it down off the shelf. It was slightly dog eared, had highlights through it and one corner had been chewed off the cover by one of our pets. I opened it and started reading.

Over the next month I gathered myself together with the aid of the book. I put into effect other coaching strategies I had learnt over the years and had used effectively on clients to aid them over roadblocks in their life. My daughter, who had been disabled by chronic fatigue for 8 years, decided to go on the journey alongside me so she read the book and she had become emotionally stronger too. We were both growing and our lives were changing.

We started setting goals as to what we wanted to manifest in our lives. I started believing that I was the master of my life. I *became* the person that had the perfect house for our needs. And then, the perfect house did become available. Things were falling into place.

I began to study personal transformation in 2021, which inspired further identity shifts within myself and created more opportunities and breakthroughs, allowing me to reach more people to aid in their transformation. I moved into a state of gratitude and I even found a sense of thankfulness and peace towards my ex-partner who had set me free to become the person I truly am meant to be. It was the loss of that relationship that gave me the motivation and the permission to shine.

Since early 2021 my identity has shifted and grown. As a Chinese Medicine practitioner, I further expanded to become a Certified Health and Wellness Coach. My dedication to visualization paired with my constant learning was paying off.

By February 2022, I was a new person. I moved to a new home and completely revamped my career. I have become an international coach with transformational programs that are changing people's lives. I am a lecturer and a clinic supervisor at Australia's leading Natural Health college. With this book, I am now a published author with many more books on the horizon. I have become the grandest version of myself, the version I have always dreamed of.

BECOMING YOUR BEST SELF

So, how does this work? How do you *be* the person *today* that you want to *become* tomorrow?

Well, the experts are correct, but somewhere we lose that little spark that lights up the whole shebang. Like having the Christmas tree all decorated but the lights aren't switched on.

Visualization is great and daily visualization during a meditation is amazing to get the feeling that you are there in the future moment of your dream life. You can *feel* the slimmer, healthier, wealthier, happier you! But in most cases it ends there.

You end the session, then get ready for work, feeling your weight, your health issues and the desperation the day before payday. You have a wistful feeling when you glance at your vision board, filled with pictures of your future life. You fervently take out your intention card asking how many ways you can keep achieving that goal you have set and affirm in the mirror as you wash your hands that you are the best you can be.

Don't get me wrong- all of these things work! The tree IS decorated! But the power that lights the tree and makes it all come alive is the *identity* of the *you* that is in all of these perceived dreams! You must *keep* feeling as if you are the person in all of the above techniques all the time! After your meditation, go about your day in the persona of this future you. Make your decisions as this future you. Dress in the style of this future you. Care for yourself as this future you. Be the future you in all ways you can be.

You may feel a little foolish at first, as if you are back to being a child and playing dress-up, as that shopkeeper or superhero. You might think, "Adults don't do that!"

If you keep at it, though, if you really envision and truly embody the feeling of having achieved your goals, gradually and with intention, it will become more familiar to you. Soon you will surprise yourself as you become more comfortable with your new persona and before you know it, you will begin to make decisions automatically from this new you.

Opportunities begin to open up, mainly because now you are noticing them from this new persona, where before you would have either not noticed, or would have passed them over as too audacious.

And as this future you becomes the present you and as you implement the other actions that will help you grow like meditation, goal setting and more visualization, the *New You* grows and grows and your world begins to expand. Your life becomes the living embodiment of the vision you had held in your mind. You are quite literally creating your life.

THE BIOLOGY OF CHANGE

Change is like teaching your dog to fetch. You get your dog to sit. You get the stick and show it to him. You put it in his mouth and close his jaws around it. You jiggle it a bit so he gets the feel of the stick in his mouth and starts salivating and he closes his jaws around it spontaneously. It is a GAME. Then you take the stick out of his mouth and throw it away! He chases it as it is an automatic reaction to chase after it. Of course, getting your dog to bring it back to you as you know is a whole other ball game!

MANIFESTATION AND MERGING

During your meditation time, visualize into the future. Turn up the brightness, the volume and *experience* your future life. Imagine future scenarios. Smell the smells, feel the feels, live the life. It's just like having the stick in the dog's mouth. Then "throw" the picture out there and leave it in the future. Come back and live your day knowing that the future is yours, the same as working on a Friday and knowing that you are going home to your favorite dinner and best company that night.

The secret is staying in the *identity* of that future you. As you already know, the subconscious can't differentiate between images and reality, so with extreme emotion it will take that as the Truth.

WHY DOES IT WORK?

When we go to sleep at night, our mind goes about processing the things that happened during the day. The brain sorts and stores information. The brain has a system of storing important information so that it will be easier to access in the future. When your brain comes across your visualization of your preferred identity scene with all its attached emotion, the strong emotions indicate to your brain that this information is important so the pathways to this information are made strong.

The way this works is that the brain uses a process called myelination to coat the pathways of information that we need to access frequently. The neural pathways are coated more and more as you utilize the information more frequently. When you visualize often, your brain comes across the same information and it begins to coat the pathways to this information so that it is easier to access. This myelination causes the chemical electrical impulses to travel faster down the neuron to this identity location and it quickly becomes the "norm", the go-to pathway.

This is how we change our identity. Myelination of neural pathways is the key.

It can happen by habituation of a task. An example of this is where an athlete practices shooting hoops over and over. The constant practice allows the impulses to travel along the pathways so frequently and this gives the neural pathways the myelination needed to make the pathway strong and the action automatic. This is the reason that practice makes perfect. It is the myelination of the pathways that creates expertise.

It can also happen from intense emotion. We often see after a traumatic event where the neural pathway is quickly and heavily myelinated in a compressed period of time. This can result in Post Traumatic Stress Disorder (PTSD). Under a microscope these impulses are seen as little chemical electrical particles of light traveling down the neural pathways. You have the choice on which pathway those chemical-electrical light particles take. You choose where to channel your Light. This determines what expression of light you will bring to the planet.

We all have an infinite ability to change because we have billions of neural pathways that we can configure for a desired outcome. The reality is that less than 5% of what we do each day is original. This is because our brain seeks to conserve energy. Since the myelinated pathways are the path of least resistance, we tend to act upon those familiar thoughts. In order to create change, we must create new pathways and we do this by visualizing new ways of being and learning what we need to learn to get there. This is the way that we rewire our brains.

This is what Deepak Chopra means when he says we have infinite possibilities. Most people limit their light. Most people limit their hopes and dreams. Don't let that be you. Pick your Christmas tree, decorate it and then *light it up!*

Thoughts become things. If you see it in your mind, you will hold it in your hand.

~ BOB PROCTOR

ABOUT THE AUTHOR

Dr. Caitlyn Brightmon is the co-founder of Soulinspire. She is a Registered Chinese Medicine Practitioner, certified Mindvalley Holobody and Transformation coach, Reiki and Qigong Master, Bowen, Acutonics and Resonance Practitioner of over 25 years.

Her passion is transforming people's lives in all ways (mentally, emotionally, spiritually and physically), by aligning their Values with their vision, removing resistance and creating heart centered habits to maximize their potential, transforming physically and emotionally to create the life they deserve.

She is a Dingo (Australia's wolf) advocate, guardian to 4 pure dingoes, mother and grandma. She loves to bellydance and is curious about how this universe works and how those in this universe ticks.

Contact Information:
Website: www.soulinspire.net
LinkedIn: http://linkedin.com/in/caitlyn-brightmon
Facebook: Facebook.com/caitlynbrightmon.official
Instagram:Instagram.com/caitlynbrightmon.official

Visualization and belief in a pattern of reality activate the creative power of realization.

~A. L. Linall Jr.

The third stage of enlightenment happens when you have become capable of finding the inner being ... this is what tantra calls Mahamudra, the great orgasm, what Buddha calls Nirvana, what Lao Tzu calls Tao and what Jesus calls the kingdom of God. You have found the door to God. You have come home.

~Swami Dayan Giten

CHAPTER 5

THE COAT RACK

CONNECTING TO AUTHENTICITY BY HANGING UP IDENTITIES

by Andre Roggy

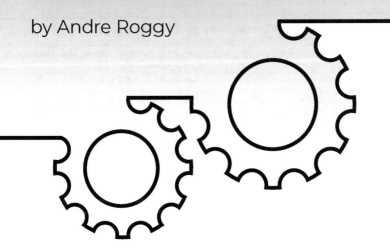

TOPIC:	Clarifying Identity
TOOL:	The Coat Rack
TECHNIQUE:	Connecting to authenticity by hanging up identities that you no longer want to identify with.

*Authenticity is a collection of choices that
we have to make every day.
It's about the choice to show up and be
real. The choice to be honest.
The choice to let our true selves be seen.*

~ BRENE BROWN

When I was very young, I smiled and laughed at almost anything, I unabashedly sang out loud at the drop of a hat and dreamed of Disney magic. There were fears, too, for sure; the Disney films I watched fed into this because of the story lines around getting lost, braving the great unknown or having to face massive obstacles.

A voraciously inquisitive and dreamy child, I found myself exploring and experiencing the world up close. I was particularly creative. I loved to create and I used anything and everything I could find in my explorations of the world. I remember discovering a tube of baby cream which decided to smear all over mirrors and cabinets like a Jackson Pollock enthusiast at age 3. When I got older, it was outdoor fun where I could make mud in the backyard and imagine I was a powerful wizard, controlling the elements of the earth. Older still, I would spend hours playing with Legos creating the most amazing, fantastical castles and structures I could imagine. I loved to play.

When it came to people, however, I found myself painfully awkward and unimaginative. People I couldn't crack. I found it especially uncomfortable around my peers. I didn't know how to interact with and navigate the social climate, as my family was not exactly very active in the community. It didn't help that I always felt so "special" that I was hyper-conscious of every move I made, too. I craved interaction and acceptance, but hadn't a clue how to unglue my flower from the wall.

Adding in the dynamics within my family I had an emotionally and often physically absent father who I never felt like I could connect with. I was different from my siblings and that feeling of being other kept me from feeling super close to them. I didn't feel like I could be myself.

And thus, as a survival mechanism, I learned the art of performance and people-pleasing. I would be the wunderkind, the "good boy," the "one that we don't have to worry about 'making it.'" I tried on this persona within my family in order to earn this identity and status. I also tried to display this new hyper achieving persona to my peers but it was met with mixed effect. Kids can be jealous or shunning when someone outperforms them.

It was a delicate balance that I learned. I became a chameleon. I changed my persona depending on who I was around. I deftly learned how to juggle the respect of my parents and other adults while also avoiding getting total beat downs on the school playground — if not to fit in, at least to be safe.

I became truly proud of my chameleon skills, adapting to my circumstances. I learned how important clothing is from an embarrassing moment in preschool when I chose to wear lederhosen to my graduation. I remember the reactions of those around me and this taught me that I had to wear clothing that allowed me to fit it. I began to pay attention to my appearance and focused on buying the coolest, most up to date clothing I could find.

If my camouflaging skills provided me any relief or belonging, it was only temporary or superficial. In the world of childhood, there are certain experiences that show you whether you truly fit in or not and in those moments, it was always clear to me that I did not fit in. I remember in gym class when the kids were picking teams, I was always picked last. It hurt me and cemented my lifelong feeling of not belonging anywhere.

I knew there had to be a better way to acceptance and peace. I struggled to find it. It took me years of struggling with failures in jobs, goals and especially personal relationships for me to search out the best way to find love. My journey towards finding a way to proudly express my authenticity as well as allow people to do the same has been one fraught with many ups and downs.

I became a seeker, traveling and experiencing the outside world to help define me. I sought out the best teachers and gurus I could, learning from them all. I searched and searched and searched until I realized that the answer I was seeking was within me all the time. I had all the answers that I needed, I just hadn't realized it.

After all of my endless seeking, I learned that I've been here all along, beneath and connected to my layers of identities.

Think of the time, energy and money I could have saved had I known! But alas, we can only know once we have taken the journey. I know now that this journey of life is not about what is out there but what is about what is in here. Inside each one of us we have all we need to feel loved and to feel like we belong here on this earth. And once you realize this, you are set free.

IDENTITIES

So, let's take a moment to look at identities and their trappings.

Identities give us a place to belong, a group to be a part of, an identification that gives us key descriptive information about ourselves and the world around us. The fallacy lies in how superficial our identities truly are, even the ones we identify so strongly with. We often think of our identities and say "this is totally me" like it's some perfectly attuned horoscope, but closer examination shows that those identities are just carefully constructed facades that we wear like armor, protecting our vulnerable selves from the harsh world we live in.

We create these false identities and they make us end up feeling like we are 2-D characters rather than full-fledged, real beings. We go through our lives presenting our identities to others and we shield who we really are. We go on dates and get into relationships and often, the other person still doesn't know who we are even after the wedding vows!

I lay some of the blame on the present-day speed with which we navigate life and the propensity to try to make split-second diagnoses and categorize our interactions and people around us. For example, walking past someone on the street, we look at their outward appearance such as age, gender expression, hair and skin color, clothing choices, gait and mannerisms, perceived mood and expression, as well as how they are interacting with others and ourselves. We assess so that we can determine if they are friend or foe. If we are safe around them. We judge to protect ourselves.

When we look at someone else, we are also looking so we can determine whether they have something we want (transactional value), as well as assessing whether we are better or worse by comparison (self-validation).

The quickness with which we tick off a list of items to determine how we handle someone or something is considered efficient, but it's at the expense of knowing the authentic nature and nuances of the actual person before us.

My point in stating all this is the idea that today's societies and the humans within them are generally shirking such thoughts and simply donning their identities, making snap judgments so they can move along to make more, all for seeming efficiency and happiness. But what I believe happens in reality is that we constantly walk around with such weight and constriction upon our natural selves, hampering our innately beautiful beings and existence, never truly revealing ourselves.

We set ourselves up for stress by worrying about wearing the best outfit, donning the most youthful, attractive face, flaunting the latest trend or title and acquiring the most assets or things. We define ourselves by our identities so that they can gain us validation for existing, when the truth is, we all are existing regardless of whatever identities we have or don't have.

We all have a unique array of identities at any given moment. They are us and yet they are only part of the story. They are labels. They are aspects. They are not the product or core beneath. And, at the epicenter — if we go deep — we can all say, "I am." Not because of what we do or the fact that we think (sorry, Descartes), but because we exist.

These identities harm us on a mental and emotional level which in turn, affects us physically. It is important to strip away all of the identities we have assumed so that we can go back to the true, radically authentic selves we are underneath all facades.

So, let's get "meta."

Metaphysics is the contemplation on the origin of being, what really is and isn't and orientation within and without existence. It can encompass thoughts such as "what is the meaning of life," "what is my purpose," and "does a higher power/God exist?"

I propose that thinking outside our perceivable, tangible knowledge and identities and instead connecting to our core existence, we can inhabit our natural springs of joy, pure love and abundant peace; and, from there, we can create, interact within and without and truly express ourselves. It is when we express the wholeness of who we are that we are able to become healthy mentally and emotionally. By becoming our true selves, we integrate body, mind and spirit and this translates into sound physical health.

As I worked to become the best version of myself, I learned many different techniques but the best one I have discovered is The Coat Rack Exercise. It has worked for me and it is my hope that it will work for you as well.

THE COAT RACK EXERCISE

The goal of this process is to hang up as many identities as you can for a short time. This allows you to become more conscious of what you choose so that you can feel more self-creative and determined rather than imposed upon.

Disrobing the numerous layers we wear is a tremendous experience. The lightness, the openness, the sense of oneness with life, joy and love is liberating. It is like you are becoming the true essence of Self versus the egotistical self rooted in identity. And like peeling an onion, there are a number of layers down we can go. See what happens for yourself and how comfortable you are with how far you can go.

The process involves a soft, focused attention for a sustained period. It feels like a meditation as you go through the steps. You examine and then calmly disrobe and hang up identities, one at a time. A similar concept would be counting sheep to assist falling asleep; except, here the aim is to remain awake, the identities replace the sheep, the questions you ask replace the jumping and counting and the fence or moon becomes the receptive coat rack.

Please note, identities can be obvious or less so — usually the deeper we go, the more abstract and general they become, such as:

- Names we use or we're given
- Roles we play (e.g. child, parent, sibling, worker, friend)
- Groups we are a part of (including cultures and our species)
- The physical self (body) and senses
- The perceived self (the mind and our self judgments)
- The perceived non-self (others, society, life)
- Things we've experienced or learned
- Specific emotions we closely identify with
- Fears, regrets, worries, longings and aspirations (specific and general)
- Space (location, proximity to others and things)
- Time (past, present, future)

Play with what ways you mentally shed your identities and go with the flow, like you are just continually and calmly speaking to yourself and sensing (seeing/feeling/imagining) the identity lifting off of you. You can place it on whatever you imagine, a coat rack or floating off into the ethos.

Remember, these identities aren't going away permanently, just by your own choosing for your own determined amount of time.

QUESTIONS

Questions are the vehicle or movement for the identities. They are the best way to get the mind to open and release rather than grasp tightly. General sample questions to get you started are:

1. Who am I without [being] _____?
2. What would it be like if I let go of [being] _____?
3. For just the time being, can I set aside [being] _____?

Try any combination of these questions or your own. If you feel that your mind is holding onto a particular identity, don't fret. Stay in the calm focus as much as you can, as there's no pressure to do so, ultimately. Try the stuck identity sequentially with different questions as if you were an expert massage therapist gently working a muscle knot. Or, come back to it after trying a few other identities and see if it will shift then. Either way, take note of this particularly clingy identity and do your own introspection. This might also be a point you may want to discuss with a trusted friend, coach or counselor.

I hope you find "The Coat Rack" both a liberating and soul-satisfying activity, a chance to really inhabit the authentic, real you. The process allows you to shed the identities you no longer want to hold onto so that you can connect with and create a new identity that works for you and where you are in life today.

For myself, I find this "meta" process helps me tap into that youthful frivolity and wonder I had before I was indoctrinated into worldly expectations and survival. I'm more me than I was for most of my life.

"The Coat Rack" is something I've coined to be a helpful visual, metaphorical process/meditation. Deeply indebted to Eastern methodologies and practitioners, I developed and packaged it together due to learning from the likes of Deepak Chopra and Mooji, the philosophies and practices of Zen Buddhism, Hinduism and more.

Only the truth of who you are, if realized, will set you free.

~ ECKHART TOLLE

ABOUT THE AUTHOR

André Roggy is a certified coach, international speaker, youth mentor, activist and writer. Being particularly passionate about the topics of conscious living, authenticity and holistic and mental health, he is eager to dialogue and promote true connections within our individual selves, amongst each other and with the world. André is currently dancing and singing to his own tune in New York City, USA.

Contact Information:
Email: aroggy@gmail.com
Linkedin: https://www.linkedin.com/in/andre-roggy

Only the truth of who you are, if realized, will set you free.

~Eckhart Tolle

CHAPTER 6

RADICAL AUTHENTICITY: THE GATEWAY TO TRANSFORMATION

by Alexandra Merlo

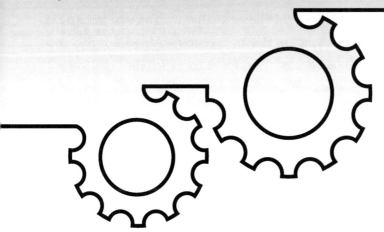

TOPIC:	Mental Health
TOOL:	Radical Acceptance
TECHNIQUE:	Embracing all of who you are by facing the deepest truths about yourself and then living from those truths and embodying the most radically authentic version of yourself.

If you trade your authenticity for safety,
you may experience the following:
Anxiety, depression, eating disorders, addiction, rage, blame,
resentment and inexplicable grief.

~ BRENÉ BROWN

When you experience any or all of the conditions Brené mentioned above, it is your body's emergency warning system letting you know that there is a gap between who you currently are and who you desire to be on the deepest level.

In this chapter I will share how I came to find Radical Authenticity to be the key, the gateway to lasting transformation. I will also share some of the tools and lessons that have helped me discover who the real me is. I am super vulnerable here, totally raw and real because it is my deepest wish that you are able to take something from this and implement it in your own life. I want you to experience the intense freedom of being aligned with your soul's purpose because it is only by aligning our head, heart and hand that you can walk the path of your dreams.

Have you ever been in a dark place? I have. I have been there. I have felt feelings of self hate, uselessness, worthlessness. I have felt like I don't belong, like I'm not wanted. I have felt like I was a burden, had nothing to offer and was a drag on the people I loved. This ultimately led me to wishing I wasn't here anymore. I was like that for a very long time. But it all changed a couple of years ago and now, I'm a published author, an international coach and a badass business woman!

The point I am making is this. I see you. I know what you're feeling and I know there is a way through it. I am not special! If I can do this, if I can go from wishing I would not wake up each morning to now jumping out of bed each day, excited to live my passion then *so can you*!

Sure it can seem hard at times, even impossible. But there was a time in your life where you didn't know how to walk or talk or even brush your teeth. These things once seemed like an impossible task but now, you do them with ease. Just as you learned how to do those things, you will learn how to live your passion.

I believe that you are reading these words right now for a reason. It is a sign. A sign that you are ready to change, that you are ready to embrace the best version of yourself. In fact, I want you to make a commitment to yourself right now. A commitment to go on this journey of health and well-being. You can do it. You can.

So make this commitment to yourself, "I will show up for myself in this moment right now and be open to the possibility that I have the power to change my life."

Okay, you have made the commitment, are you ready to dive in? Let's go.

Let me take you back to 2020, the year that all of our lives changed. The year the pandemic came and the entire world shut down. The year we were all in our homes, not able to see one another or go out or to do anything other than sit and wait to see what would happen.

This was the year that my entire life changed. The first half of the year I would describe as possibly the worst months of my life. I had been living with chronic fatigue as well as a neurological disability for 8 years. I was unable to work, I was unable to live independently. I was completely lost.

I had no sense of who I was or what I was capable of doing. I wasn't even sure I could do anything at all. I was angry, depressed and resentful. It felt very bleak indeed.

One day, a dear friend contacted me and they really needed my help. Helping my friend brought me a sense of purpose and fulfillment. It felt good to be able to support her. During that time period, I was able to distract myself from my own problems by focusing on helping my friend.

Once my friend's situation improved, it was back to the same situation. I was feeling like I was drifting back into a dark place. At this point, my living circumstances changed and my mother and I were forced to find a new home. We struggled to find a suitable place for the two of us and our various pets, five dogs and a cat.

Around this time my mother shared a book with me that completely changed my outlook. The book shared lessons on manifestation, affirmations and the idea of our thoughts shaping our reality. I was desperate and needed something to cling to so this book became my bible. I read parts of it every day and something happened. My view of the world around me shifted. I started seeing things in a more positive way and it felt like a lot more positive things were happening.

This brought me to the beginning of 2021 which is when I started my journey of personal development in earnest. My living situation changed again, to a much better place and I was starting to feel better. I was in a better place in many ways, but I still wasn't happy. I didn't feel like I was fully myself and I still had no idea what to do with my life or even if I could do anything with my life. My days mostly consisted of watching television or pretending to support my mother with her business.

I had been working with a psychologist for ten years at this point and they suggested that I return to school. They mentioned they thought that I would make an amazing psychologist if I were able to do the years of study and then sustain the workload. I knew that was a non-starter. I had very little motivation and I doubted that I could go back to school for the years it would take to get my degree.

That was when my mother mentioned coaching. Honestly, I didn't even know what coaching was, apart from that actors and athletes use them. Then there are life coaches and my belief at that time was that they were just scam artists. Weren't they? Well perhaps some of them are, but after doing some research I discovered that there are coaches for everything.

As I researched coaching, I had a revelation. I discovered that I had been coaching in some capacity for years. I would often help my friends, family and colleagues with their lives, with their issues. There were so many times I remembered where I had helped them find solutions to problems or challenges that they were facing. As I reflected on this, I had an even bigger revelation, a life changing revelation. I realized that those moments when I was helping my friends and family members were the moments where I felt like I was the most fulfilled. I suddenly understood my life's mission. I was a coach!

I was super excited so I decided to take some trainings to learn how to be the best coach I could be. I undertook training with an incredible organization and have learnt so much about how I can best help people with all areas of life and beyond that, I learned a lot about myself. It has been and continues to be an incredible journey, but at the same time it generated a paralyzing fear in me.

You see, I still wasn't being honest with who I was. I didn't like myself, I was afraid of being myself, I was confused, sad and frustrated. So I found what I loved doing but it didn't make me happy. Not fully. Something was holding me back. I had to learn how to be myself.

But how can I be myself? How could I tell the deepest truths about myself? And what would happen if I did?

Would everything that I had been working on disappear?

So many thoughts swirled in my head. Perhaps coaching others would help me to eventually just become happy. Maybe if I am helping others, I will feel good about myself?

Unfortunately, that isn't how it works.

So there I was. I had started a journey of doing what I was meant to be, I knew my mission in life and I was passionate about it but I was still feeling like crap. At this point I had started my training as a holistic wellness coach and one of the first exercises was an exercise called the Body Relationship Journey.

The first time I did this exercise I had a revelation. You see, I had always struggled with my gender identity. From a young age I knew I was in the wrong body, but I didn't have the vocabulary to express how I was feeling. Through my teens I fought against it and pretended to be the stereotypical boy. I don't think I did a good job considering how much I was bullied. Then, when I was 18, I shared my truth with my mother but I quickly became scared of the idea of being transgender.

I had conflicting beliefs about it and would often pray that I would either miraculously wake up in the right body or that I wouldn't wake up at all. I hated my body for being wrong and I realized in this moment that I had subconsciously and perhaps consciously at times, been sabotaging my body. I hadn't been taking care of my body at all. Suddenly, I realized that my body wasn't trying to sabotage me, it was just trying to be the best support for me it could be.

I was the one sabotaging it! Bad food, no movement, negative thoughts and words. I wasn't living a healthy life. I wasn't honoring my body. I decided I had to do something to change things. I was committed to becoming the very best version of myself. I started with the body relationship journey exercise.

THE BODY RELATIONSHIP JOURNEY

The Body Relationship Journey is a great exercise. You draw a timeline of your life, one line straight across the middle with your life plotted out by years. Then, above the line, you place all the high points in your life from the standpoint of your health and your relationship with your body and below the line you place all the low points throughout your life in relation to your body. Was it in a positive state or a negative state and what was happening in your life at the time? It is an insightful process that can uncover patterns and clues to who you are and where you might want to be.

Soon after completing this exercise and continuing on my own coaching journey a big "a-ha" moment happened. I could not continue to hide who I am if my purpose is to help others accept and embrace who they truly are.

So I did it.

I told myself that from that moment I am Alex the woman. The woman I had always been but pretended I wasn't because I thought it wasn't who my loved ones wanted me to be or I was afraid of what they might think. I knew that I wasn't happy pretending to be someone that I'm not, so how much worse can being honest be? So I decided to be fully, totally, radically authentic about who I really am.

I know that it can be a vastly different story for many people depending on your background or culture, some would lose their closest family and friends by embracing their authentic self.

And that doesn't just apply to the LGBTQIA+ community. It applies to people who want to follow a different career path to what their parents wanted and people who want to stand up for issues that don't align with their family or culture. It can be anyone and anything. Maybe you grew up with your parents always wanting you to become a lawyer and off you went to law school and you were miserable because you always wanted to be a teacher but you don't want to disappoint your family. It can truly be anything.

As I thought about being fully me, I knew I needed something to help keep the fear at bay. I needed to find something that kept me focused on being authentic. I needed a tool to help me be free of judgment from myself and my perceived judgment from others.

MINDSET

This was a real fear. I used to assume that people laughing on the other side of a shopping center, who couldn't even see me, were laughing at me.

Why? Exactly, why do we let this story run in our mind that is so negative? Or even worse, why do we believe it?

Well, I have come to learn that our mind doesn't know the difference between what is real and what is imagined. The mind cannot tell what is the truth and what is a lie. If our minds only accepted the truth then everyone on the planet would have the same beliefs, we would all know with 100% certainty that the earth is flat and that all birds have gone extinct and what we see in the sky and trees are just government controlled drones. By the way, I do not believe these things.

So if our mind doesn't know the truth from lies, then it stands to reason that some of our beliefs are not technically true.

For example, have you ever reminisced on a memory with a family member who was there with you at that time and when you shared your memory of that moment your family member had a different experience entirely? That's because we tell ourselves stories and this shapes our view of the world around us.

FREEDOM STATEMENTS

This brings me to the second concept I want to share with you. The idea of creating Freedom Statements. Freedom Statements are statements that you choose to live by. I encourage you to try them and perhaps embrace them in your own life. Here are my freedom statements that I have chosen to live by:

You are under no obligation to be who you were 5 minutes ago. And what other people think about you is none of your business and has nothing to do with you.

Why did I share these Freedom Statements with you? Because they are true of course, but more often than not we believe the complete opposite. How many people do you know, you might even be one of them, who take a certain path in life and then hold yourself back from a better, more fulfilling path because you "already invested in this path", or "trained in that profession," or think "what will my husband/wife/partner think?" Or "my parents won't like it if I change". You see we put so much value on what other people think and to make matters worse we even put value on what dead people think. "Grandma would be turning over in her grave!"

This is what tradition is, tradition is peer pressure from dead people. But what if you chose to value what you wanted and what you know is right above all other opinions? You know the saying, "opinions are like arseholes, everyone has one". But let me ask you this. Do you poop out of anyone else's arsehole? Okay maybe not the best analogy but you get my point. You can make the choice right now to stop living by other peoples standards and start, just start, to take action on a path you create.

You are not defined by your past choices. Just because you studied accounting when you left school does not mean that is the only path for you, if you want to be a veterinarian you can be, if you allow yourself the freedom to choose. Which leads to this idea that we are subconsciously waiting for approval or permission to live our lives.

The most scientific way I can explain this is that when you focus on something and keep repeating a message to yourself, inside your brain there is a neurological network forming around that message and over-time, especially if you repeat it often enough over time, that neurological pathway becomes wrapped with a substance called myelin. Now myelin actually insulates the neurological pathway so that information can travel down that path several times faster than a path without the insulation of myelin, up to 100 times faster in fact. Now if you are repeating a negative statement about yourself or repeating a false belief that you cannot live the life you desire, your brain believes that and makes that belief an in-formation superhighway. Now, your brain is powerful, you know this, so powerful in fact that once that belief is nicely ingrained and myelinated it will seek to solidify this externally in the physical world and make that belief your reality.

So for me what happened was that because I didn't have the body I wanted I started telling myself that my body was the problem. I would tell myself that my body was broken, that something was wrong with me, that I'm unlovable, disgusting. Over time what happened was that my reality reflected my belief, I gained weight; I developed a disability, I isolated myself from anyone who showed an interest in me on any level and I made true what I was saying.

But the exciting thing is that it works both ways! So if you tell yourself you are beautiful, loveable, you are ENOUGH, you are smart, capable, successful, that you can choose your own path, that you can achieve any-thing you set your mind to, what happens is that your brain will believe these messages and start insulating these pathways with myelin and before you know it you have your reality reflecting those messages. Self praise is absolutely critical to your health and happiness.

So with these gems I was able to start my path of authenticity and it has radically changed my life, I am following a path that I determine, I get to smile knowing I am doing what I love and I am surrounded by acceptance for who I am including acceptance from myself which, lets face it, is the only acceptance I need. And don't get me wrong, I am still on a journey, I have ups and downs and I too will continue to grow and learn for the rest of my life. There is no destination in life where you suddenly don't have to keep growing, there is no magical end point. So take the pressure off yourself, take it one step at a time and if I can leave you with one final piece of wisdom, find a coach to be in your corner and on your team as you do it. I have never achieved anything in my life without some form of support and there is no shame whatsoever in asking for help, but quite often we ask the wrong people. So find someone who encourages you, inspires you, challenges you and allows you the space to find your own solutions.

I am so grateful for the opportunity to share with you why Radical Authenticity is the Gateway to Transformation and how through that you can live the life of your dreams. I welcome your feedback and your stories of transformation and self acceptance should you wish to share them. If you would like more information regarding me or my business, Soulinspire® and the incredible services that we provide, please feel free to send an email to support@soulinspire.net or visit our website at www. soulinspire.net.

I wish you the best of luck on your journey to Extraordinary Health. Love, Hope, Dreams.

Authentically,
Alex

The privilege of a lifetime is to become who you truly are.
~ CARL JUNG

ABOUT THE AUTHOR

Alexandra Merlo is a Holistic Transformation Coach & Co-Founder of Soulinspire. She is a Mindvalley Certified Holobody Coach, RTT Practitioner & Certified Hypnotherapist.

Alex is a transgender woman and is passionate about helping other women and members of the global LGBTQIA+ community master their mindset and realize their fullest potential.

Alex spent years plagued by fear, shame, guilt and self rejection before deciding to accept her authentic self and live her passion. Now Alex is unapologetically herself and lives each day to see others do the same for themselves.

Alex is also passionate about animals, being the custodian of 4 Dingoes (Australia's wolf), a tech connoisseur, a rom-com lover and marvel MCU nerd.

Contact Information:
Website: www.soulinspire.net
LinkedIn: linkedin.com/in/alexandramerloofficial
Facebook: facebook.com/alexandramerlo.official
Instagram: instagram.com/alexandramerlo.official

**Movement is a medicine for creating change
in a person's physical, emotional and mental states.**

~Carol Welch

CHAPTER 7

THE ACE OF CUPS

by Amrys Wang

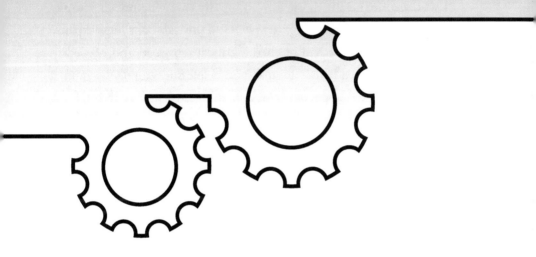

TOPIC:	Mindset
TOOL:	Self Love and Intentional Movement
TECHNIQUE:	Take care of yourself by filling your cup first. Take care of your physical, emotional and mental health through self care practices like self love and intentional movement. Fill your Ace of Cups.

Until you value yourself, you won't value your time.
Until you value your time, you will not do anything with it.

~ M. SCOTT PECK

In 2020, I was struggling with a constrictor knot in my head. I was burnt out emotionally, physically and mentally.

As an animal welfare advocate and community volunteer for several years, I was giving to everyone but myself. I was giving all my time and energy to everyone who needed help but never even considered putting myself on the list.

I was also financially drained from blindly throwing myself into my animal rescue work. I was unable to say *no* and this came at a huge expense to my own well-being. I had reached a critical crossroad and needed to change the way I lived before anguish and helplessness totally consumed me. On the outside, I appeared calm and collected but deep inside I was drowning, gasping for air. Maybe you've been there?

I knew something needed to change. I realized that my mind was overwhelmed, I was emotionally drained. I resolved to do something, anything, to create a better life for myself. My quest of self-discovery and spiritual awakening had begun.

I decided to immerse myself in personal transformation. I enrolled in the Tony Robbins' *Unleash The Power Within* virtual event which was a real game changer for me. There were many aha moments for me throughout the event. My main takeaway was that I needed to change my mindset. This insight came to me when Tony Robbins shared a study which highlighted the power of the mind over the body.

The study revolved around a group of female hotel room attendants working in seven different hotels. They were measured on physiological health variables affected by exercise. Group A were told that their work cleaning hotel rooms was good exercise and that their level of activity satisfied the Surgeon General's recommendations for an active lifestyle. Group B were not given this information. The hotel room attendants were told not to change anything. They were to maintain their current levels of activity.

Four weeks later, the hotel room attendants gathered to be retested on a variety of health markers. There were significant improvements in the health markers in the Group A attendants. This was interesting because Group A was the group that was told that their work was considered an active lifestyle. They perceived themselves to be getting significantly more exercise than before simply by being told that their levels of activity at work qualified as a high level of exercise. As a result, Group A showed a decrease in weight, blood pressure, body fat, waist-to-hip ratio and body mass index. Group B had no change. These results supported the hypothesis that exercise affects health in part or in whole via the placebo effect. (Crum, Alia J. and Ellen J. Langer. 2007. Mindset matters: Exercise and the placebo effect. Psychological Science 18, no. 2: 165-171.)

This study intrigued me. It made me see the connection between what I was thinking and feeling (my mindset) and my physical health. I was shocked that a person's beliefs could have this much effect on their health, it was a true revelation. I finally understood the connection between body, mind and emotions for the very first time.

I examined my own physical and emotional state. I realized that both were a mess. I knew in that instant that I needed to change my mindset. I needed to learn how to take care of myself both physically and mentally. I had to get my emotional life in order. I understood very clearly that the best way to do that was to love myself enough to take the time to take care of myself, to fill myself up.

I came up with the idea that I needed to learn how to F.L.Y.—First Love Yourself, to fill my cup first.

This was such an alien concept to me since I had spent most of my life blindly following what everyone else was doing, blindly following what I had been taught. I had been living by a bunch of bullshit rules, or "brules" as some people call them. A brule is a rule that we adopt to simplify our understanding of the world. It is a rule that we adopt so we can play it safe, so we can meet other people's expectations of us. Some common brules are: Hard Work equals success; Money is evil; Love is painful; Humans are evil.

One of the brules I was living by was the belief that I did not deserve to be happy while others were suffering. It was a brule I had lived by for my entire life. I had always felt so much responsibility for those around me, for the suffering in the world and this prevented me from finding happiness for myself. I bought into the idea that if other people were suffering, then I had to suffer too. I decided to break away from this brule which allowed me to drop the heavy emotional burden I had always carried. Releasing that brule had set me free.

At the time I was assessing all the different rules I lived by, I discovered that I was scared and terrified of change. I knew I must change if I was to break away from this quagmire and move into a life of ease and flow so I dug deep and found the courage to take action daily. It felt super uncomfortable, but I chose to embrace discomfort. Once I did this, a switch flipped inside my head.

A deep seated hunger was released and I began to consume as much information on personal development as my left brain allowed. Eventually I learned to relax and give my right brain the freedom to explore. I let my intuition guide me to open my heart to infinite possibilities and most importantly, I learned that loving myself first is the key to unlocking the door to becoming a better human being.

I loved this journey of transformation I was on. Each day I felt better, stronger and more resilient. I kept learning, I kept practicing, I kept putting the new ideas I had into practice. I began to change. My life began to change. It was incredible.

It happened for me because I took daily, consistent action. Small steps day by day until I noticed my life beginning to change. The most impactful tool I used was the technique of loving myself first, or the FLY system. It's a great system which worked for me and it can work for anyone who wants to change their mindset.

LEARNING HOW TO FLY: FIRST LOVE YOURSELF

If needed, oxygen masks will be released overhead.
To start the flow of oxygen, reach up and pull the mask
toward you, fully extending the plastic tubing.
Place the mask over your nose and mouth
and slip the elastic band over your head.
To tighten the fit, pull the tab on each side of the mask.
The plastic bag does not need to inflate when oxygen is flowing.
Be sure to secure your own mask before assisting others.

~ PRE-DEPARTURE SAFETY SPEECH

Hopefully most of us adventurers have not forgotten this pre-departure public safety announcement given on all commercial flights. This is a reminder to see to your personal safety first. To prevent you from passing out and harming yourself or others inadvertently.

This logic translates well into one's daily life. As you focus your energy towards self- improvement and start to practice daily self-care, all aspects of your life will get better, enabling you to pursue your goals with gusto. You become the best version of yourself in all ways. You will notice improvements physically, emotionally, spiritually and mentally. You will find that you can do more, be more and achieve greater impact on the world you wish to create.

Some people think self-care simply means having some personal time off, a spa day or taking a holiday. These are great self-care tips to recharge your energy but to have a long-lasting impact on your self-development, one must go deeper and practice self-love. Self-love means believing that you are worthy of love. That you deserve to have good things happen to you. To give yourself permission to be more loving and kind towards yourself. Instead of limiting yourself, open yourself up to opportunities. To learn to say NO to situations that don't uplift you. To learn to forgive yourself and let go of the past and whatever does not serve you anymore. To live with gratitude.

By consciously prioritizing self-love in your daily routine, you are creating a continuous cycle of positive emotions like joy, gratitude and love flowing into your body. These emotions will create positive changes in your brain. You will start to feel these changes and that's when the magic happens.

SHIFTING YOUR ENERGY

One of my mentors, Feng Shui master Marie Diamond, made an interesting observation of the word 'change'. The word change consists of two parts: 'ch' for 'chi' or energy and 'ange' for 'angle' or perspective. In order to change, you need to transform your energy and shift your perspective.

Everything is made up of energy. Every person, place and thing vibrates at different frequencies. When someone has a high vibrational energy that means his/her energetic frequency is emotionally positive, good and strong. Conversely, a low vibrational energy is associated with negative emotions such as suffering, fear and anger.

To find the right frequency that will raise one energetically, we need to learn how to change and finetune our energetic frequency until it resonates with our higher self, our soul. The best part is the universe loves you and wants to help you evolve into a better being. We are not alone, my friend.

There are many methods on how to achieve that but I am going to share what I believe to be at the heart of all methods: intentional movement. Setting your intention and consciously acting on it. Movement is essential in creating energetic change physically, emotionally, mentally and spiritually. To prevent misalignment, you need to take conscious action to create the change you want to become.

When people think of intentional movement, they may think of exercises like yoga, qigong or tai chi, which provide many health benefits to help connect the body and mind; heal the body and soul; gain clarity and focus; clear blocked energy; and an improved sense of well-being. These are all excellent practices that I have incorporated into my self-love toolkit.

However, I view intentional movement as even more nuanced. Everything I do when done consciously with intention is an intentional movement. To live consciously is to act consciously and to move with intention. I learnt that the fastest way to change my mood was to move my body. By changing my physiology, I could change my state of mind. Think of the time when you felt crappy and decided to go for a walk, or an invigorated run, rearranged the furniture in your living room or danced with a kitten in your arms. How did you feel after that? Having personally done all of the above, all feel pretty darned good. What's even better is that when you feel good, you're nicer to those around you too.

Since proactively introducing intentional movements of self-love into my daily life, I have found myself less reactive to events around me and I have developed more self- awareness on what triggers me. I am a lot kinder to myself now and instead of piling on the guilt for making a mistake, I review the incident, reflect on my emotional responses and make a mental note. I remind myself that now that I know better, I can do better next time. And then I release the incident energetically back to the universe and thank my guides for the lesson. A beautiful side effect of practicing self-love is what I call the Ripple Effect: those around you will feel that warm nourishing self-love emanating from your heart and will be all the richer for it.

A quick intentional movement that I like to do when I feel stuck and frustrated is to stand on an elevated (make sure it's stable) surface like a bench or table to change my perspective of the room. I straighten my posture, head high, shoulders pulled back and take slow deep breaths as I survey my kingdom with The Lion King music "Circle of Life / Nants' Ingonyama" playing. When I do this, I feel calmer and in alignment with all around me.

Now it's your turn. Try it. Can you hear the music? Is your heart stirring? Is your body feeling goosebumps? Are you standing on your chair? By changing your physiology and incorporating emotional music with your movement, you will find that your mood instantly changes. This is a great exercise because it's a reminder to always look at the world from another angle, to challenge traditional ideas and to ask better questions. It's a chance to look at yourself, at others and at situations from another perspective. It allows you to gain inspiration for a different result.

Going back to the study of the female hotel room attendants, I changed my perspective on house cleaning. Where I once hated it and felt that it was a 'chore', a waste of time but a necessary evil that I resented, I stopped using the term 'house chores' and now call it my 'Home Gratitude Routine'.

Doing my home gratitude routine allows me to find my *why*. Why I love my animals and my family. Why I want to create a healthy, clean and welcoming home environment for all humanimals.

As I vacuum, do the laundry, hang the clothes in the wardrobe, clear the cat litter boxes, walk the dog, feed and wash up after the animals, I now do so with clarity of purpose. Every intentional movement I make, I do it out of love for my 'fur'mily. I use this time to express my thanks to the universe for providing me with a beautiful safe sanctuary to care for such an amazing furmily. I am thankful that this self love ritual of taking care of my home provides me with daily teachings in perseverance, patience and unconditional love. It challenges me to become a better caregiver and human being by taking care of my home with love and gratitude. And my furmily is healthier and happier as a result. A true blessing indeed!

The best part of the Home Gratitude Routine? I get my minimum dose of physical exercise for the day and that's my win! Anything extra is a bonus! It doesn't matter what time I do my Home Gratitude as I know exactly why I am doing it and it fills my cup. I call this my Ace of Cups.

That is the power of intentional movement when serving a higher purpose from a place of no blame, no shame, just pure love from the heart. A heart that has been filled with self-love first.

It has been two years since I started this journey of self-discovery, of self-love. I am still a student learning and growing daily. I no longer identify myself as an animal welfare advocate but an animal wellness advocate. I wake up every day now and thank the universe for giving me another wonderful opportunity to serve my community with a better version of myself compared to yesterday. To fully embrace all that life has to offer. Amor Fati.

Have you filled your Ace of Cups?

Blessings Be To All.
Amrys

The unexamined life is not worth living.

~ SOCRATES

ABOUT THE AUTHOR

Amrys Wang, founder of The Raw Entrepawneur Podcast, is a dedicated Pet Longevity Junkie and cheeky Spiritual Seeker of Infinite Possibilities filled with magic and miracles.

She's on a mission to empower inspired pet parents to become conscious caregivers for humanimals. As a passionate animal wellness advocate and community volunteer, Amrys quickly suffered burnout at the expense of her own well-being; painfully realizing this was neither helping the animals she cared for nor the life she envisioned for herself.

Amrys realized that if she wanted to create positive meaningful change, she needed to learn how to F.L.Y.—First Love Yourself, by taking control of her own life starting with her health before she could help others. Amrys' journey of self-discovery and personal growth has led her to help others do the same.

Contact Info:
Website: https://TheRawEntrepawneur.com
Linktree: https://linktr.ee/therawentrepawneur
Instagram: @TheRawEntrepawneur

I challenge you to make your life a masterpiece. I challenge you to join the ranks of those people who live what they teach, who walk their talk.

~Tony Robbins

**Mastering others is strength.
Mastering yourself is true power.**

~Lao Tzu

CHAPTER 8

MINDING YOUR EMOTIONS

by Priti Shah

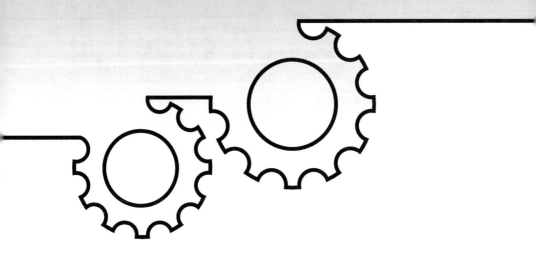

TOPIC:	Emotions and Self Love Practices
TOOL:	Getting Clear and Practicing Self Love
TECHNIQUES:	Self Reflection, Getting a Coach, Self Compassion, Journaling, and Forgiveness.

*Anything that's human is mentionable,
and anything that is mentionable can be more manageable.
When we can talk about our feelings, they become
less overwhelming, less upsetting and less scary.*

~ FRED ROGERS

I grew up not understanding much about health and wellness. I certainly didn't understand that emotional health was even part of the health equation, that's for sure. It was not until my father passed away that I began to realize exactly how much emotions have to do with healthy living.

My father passed away in October 2021. When he died, I was on autopilot for a while. My brain was in a fog. I had so many emotions coming up but I just pushed them back down. It's what I had been taught to do. I was struggling. The grief was overwhelming.

About two weeks after my father died, I began to have strange symptoms. I felt a sudden pain in my right heel, which was odd because I had not hurt myself in any way. I was having other aches and pains as well. I had no energy or stamina and I found myself depleted in every way. Climbing a short flight of stairs or walking a very short distance made me completely out of breath. I wasn't sure what was happening but looking back, I believe that it was the grief and pain of my father's passing expressing itself in my body.

I began to feel bloated as if my body were swollen. I was gaining weight quickly. My body just kept getting bigger and bigger. It was terrible but I wasn't able to do anything about it, I was suffering greatly. My health was not good and I knew something had to change. I just didn't know what. By December of 2021, my health was at an all-time low and I was at a point where I was tired of being tired, tired of being sick, tired of it all.

At this point, a lot of memories from the past began to surface and I began to feel a lot of emotions surfacing. The memories of these events in my life were bubbling up, coming into my consciousness for the very first time. They were events which I had not dealt with at the time, things I had brushed aside. These were memories which I had somehow even 'forgotten' because it was too much for me to handle at the time they happened. Suddenly, it all came tumbling back, along with the emotions attached to these events, emotions I had long suppressed. Something about my father's death had made the emotions of each of these past events begin to rise up in my mind. It all began to surface.

As this was happening, the connection was made for me. I realized that the emotions of my father's death had triggered this cascade of past emotions. I also understood that there might be a connection between my emotions and my bodily aches and pains. I began to realize that this was what people were talking about when they said that unexpressed emotions showed up in the body as some kind of pain or disease. Or, more accurately, these emotions were showing up as dis-ease.

I started to reflect on my life. I knew I had gone through different ups and downs in my life, but in terms of my health, I always thought I had been healthy until this recent bout with ill health after my father's death. In terms of my health, I considered my recent problems a new development. I decided I needed to do something about my health so I decided to watch a master class on health.

TIMELINE HEALTH JOURNEY

During the masterclass, the instructor had us do an exercise where we were to draw a timeline of our lives. We were then to determine where we had been in our lives in terms of health. We had to write the times we were in peak health above the timeline on the appropriate year and the times when we were not in great health below the line on the appropriate year. This would give us a timeline of health throughout our lives.

I did the exercise and was really surprised at what I discovered. I found that for most of my life, my health was below the line, indicating that I was in poor health or had a physical issue for much of my life. It was a shock to me. It was then that I realized that I had assumed something about my health that was untrue. I had been thinking I was healthy but the facts showed otherwise. It was a true wakeup call.

It was an interesting moment of self discovery and actually quite amusing, because it was my pursuit of a healthy life and my desire to learn how to heal naturally after my father's death which had brought me across this health workshop in the first place. It was my desire to be healthy in all ways that brought me to the program that would ultimately help me realize that I was not as healthy as I thought. I knew I needed to approach my health in a different way than I ever had before.

I began a healthy journey of transformation that has changed everything for me. I began to study health and learned many things. One of the most impactful things I learned was that emotions play a huge part in creating a healthy lifestyle. This was a true wakeup call to me because I had never considered how emotions are such a crucial aspect of health. As I learned more about it, I suddenly understood how our emotions affect every aspect of our health.

Emotions are a vital part of our lives, almost like breathing. They play such a big role in every second of our lives. There are both positive and negative emotions and every emotion in between. Every emotion affects us. For example, when you are happy, you feel great, uplifted and ready to take on the world. On the other hand, when you are sad, you feel down in the dumps. This shows us how emotions directly affect our actions and why it is so important to learn to deal with all emotions as they arise.

Although there are people who can deal with their emotions easily, there are many people who do not know how to handle the emotions at all. The vast majority of people live in cultures that do not encourage any examination of emotions at all. People are simply not taught how important emotions are and how they affect us mentally and physically too.

Imagine going through life without knowing what emotions can do. Many people go through life this way and treat the symptoms of the disease, the pain, the mental suffering, without any knowledge that it is the emotions they have to work with.

And it was the same for me too. I held on to so many emotions, not knowing how to deal with them, being affected tremendously by them and not knowing they were having any affect on my health. I simply never made the connection between my health and my emotions and this left me confused, wondering why my body was in the state it was in.

Why am I not able to move? Why isn't my body supporting me physically? Why am I gaining so much weight? Why don't I have any energy? It was a complete mystery to me. That's where I was before I did that exercise where I had to plot my health highs and lows on the chart. I simply didn't know the answers to these questions. But once I looked at my timeline and saw that my health lows always coincided with a very stressful time in my life, it all became clear. And that's when I was able to begin to turn my health around.

Maybe this resonates with you. Maybe you see yourself in this story. If you do, have faith that you can do something about it. The key is recognizing why you are in the health state you are in. Once you begin to make that connection between how you are feeling physically and how you are feeling mentally, you can begin to learn how to deal with your emotions. Once you do this, the journey of life becomes easier and better.

I spent most of my life trying to find a way to feel good, to keep my weight in a healthy zone, to have more energy. I tried to make myself healthy by exercising and dieting but nothing worked until I faced the truth about how much my body was affected by my mind. And that has been my journey since that day in December. I began to pay attention to how I was feeling and to connect it with how I was taking care of myself and things began to change.

My journey is not complete, at the time of writing this. But there are many things I have done and that I am doing as I go along. The best thing is that the path keeps opening up for me on what to do to continue my health transformation. It all started with my mindset. And here is where I will start on how to go about this journey, from what I have learnt so far.

TIPS TO MOVE TOWARDS VIBRANT HEALTH

Tip 1: Uncovering the Reason for Your Current State of Health: Getting Clear

As part of my journey towards health, I decided to study Neuro Linguistic Programming (NLP). NLP is a form of reprogramming pioneered by Richard Bandler and John Grindler wherein the practitioner helps the client to rewire beliefs within the unconscious mind. It is a process of uncovering thinking patterns in order to eliminate those that are not serving us and then create positive thinking patterns.

The first thing I learned during the training is that mindset is the key to everything. Our mindset, in turn, determines how we behave.

What is mindset? Mindset is a set of beliefs that we have about the world. Mindset encompasses what we believe about health, relationships, family, society, religion, as well as our beliefs about the world. Our mindset is made up of our perception which comes from all the people, places and things that have influenced us, everything we are surrounded by. This includes parents, siblings, extended family, neighbors, teachers, friends, media, culture and the society we are raised in. Our beliefs also come from all the things we have experienced in our lives. All of these things affect our beliefs, our perception, our mindset.

This brings up the next aspect of mindset which is our emotional state. Understanding emotions and the way that our emotions affect us is the key to everything. We need to consider how we deal with our emotions and the mindset we have about healing ourselves.

The key question to ask is, "Do I truly want to get well or have I re-signed myself to being in ill health?"

As you examine this question, think about whether you truly want to get well or if, perhaps, you want to stay ill because of the attention and care it brings you. This can be a painful question to ask and it isn't one that most people ask themselves, but if you are willing to be brave and to look inwards and be brutally honest with yourself, you may be surprised that your ill health is actually satisfying some need within you to have people care for you.

Alternatively, it could be something else underlying your behavior such as that your mind and body are protecting you against something and somehow, being unwell is somehow more beneficial. This is not a deliberate thing but a failsafe mechanism of the body and mind.

Examining behaviors and then going deeper to understand the belief system underlying these behaviors can have a huge impact on the health transformation journey. This is true for everyone. We all have unconscious beliefs that affect our behavior and as we begin to uncover these beliefs, we can finally get to the root cause of our behavior. This is when true change can occur. This act of uncovering deep seated perceptions will determine the success or failure of the journey.

Tip 2: Self-love: Compassion Towards Yourself

If you really want to get well, the next thing to address is how you treat yourself. It is essential to be kind and compassionate to yourself as you begin to change your patterns. This process can be emotional so it is imperative that you give time to yourself to incorporate what you are learning so that you can truly heal.

The journey is like peeling an onion. Because we are working with emotions here, until one layer gets peeled, you don't know what the next layer holds. And as you work through these issues and emotions, there will be times when something comes up that is unexpected. Allow time for these layers to be peeled back and understood. Don't try to push too hard or too fast. Let it be a deliberate process.

I had to learn this the hard way. I remember that on that day in December when I decided to change that I wanted nothing more than to be instantly cured. As I began to work on myself, I understood that it was not going to happen overnight, I also learned how important it was to be patient with myself and to tune into what I really needed.

As I was going through my journey, a colleague and friend told me that I should look to others to help me, to support me and to encourage me. I thought about it and realized how right he was. I sought out help and it was that support that has been essential to my growth. At times on my journey when I felt immobilized and unable to do anything, it was the people who were supporting me that kept me afloat.

So, love yourself enough to get help! Ask for it. If offered, graciously accept it from wherever you can get it. These supporters will help you to stay the course until you are ready to take the next step. Ultimately, of course, you must take action yourself in order to truly move forward, however, having loving people around you who are encouraging you is essential.

Tip 3: Self-love: Get a Coach or Therapist

A great way to move forward is to get a coach or a therapist. If you are ready to move towards your goals, a coach can be essential to help you clarify your goals as well as to keep you accountable. Having a coach has helped me move forward and has been instrumental in my progress towards the healthy lifestyle I imagine.

If you are truly struggling to understand why you can't create change or if you have traumatic events in your past that you have not dealt with, it would be wise to consider getting a therapist. They can help you to work through your emotions around the event and guide you in techniques that will help you to deal with the issues that caused those emotions. As you come to terms with your past and your issues get resolved, the emotions which settled themselves into your body and showed up as a disease, or pain, or suffering of some kind, will start to release and your body will start moving back into a healthier state.

Tip 4: Journaling and Writing for Clarity

There are various tools and techniques which can help you on your healing journey.

> *Journaling:* One of the best ways to gain clarity is through journaling. You can journal in a dedicated journaling document or if you prefer to write, you can purchase a beautiful journal to write your thoughts. You could even simply record your thoughts on your phone, which would become an audio journal. There are programs that can convert voice to text if you find that you want to have a written copy of your thoughts. Remember, it's content, not format, that matters.

When you begin to journal, allow whatever is ready to flow out to simply flow out. Don't try to edit yourself or write perfectly. Don't censor yourself. You can use traditional writing by formatting it in full paragraphs or you can simply jot down short sentences. Sometimes, it's just a word that you need to write down. Allow yourself the freedom to simply write, to get those thoughts out of your head and onto the paper. A great way to start is to make a list of things you have on your mind, topics you want to explore and use this list as a starting point. Use this list to pick a topic from your list and simply start by writing down what you are feeling.

> *Letter Writing:* Another option would be to write a letter to someone who is occupying your thoughts. Allowing yourself to get the thoughts out of your head will help you to gain clarity around your feelings about the person. You can write a letter to someone you had a difficult relationship with in the past or someone that you feel harmed you. You might want to write a letter to someone who is sick or has passed away. The main thing when you write the letter is to allow yourself the freedom to write whatever you need to write. Let all the emotions come out, even if the emotions are negative ones. Remember, feeling happiness, sadness, joy, anger or even fear are all completely and utterly normal.

This technique was tremendously helpful for me when my father passed away, since his passing was unexpected and sudden. It affected me in a way I could not have imagined. When working on my grief with a grief counselor, I was advised to write a letter to him and to pour out all my heart's feelings. I was encouraged to write it all… the good, the bad, everything. For me, the most impactful thing I wrote was those things that I had not said to him, the words I had wanted to say but could no longer say. It was healing in a deep way and helped me to feel connected to my father even though he was gone.

The reason that journaling and writing letters works is that when things are put on paper, you gain perspective. Writing gives relief, it eases your emotions, helps you to acknowledge things and ultimately helps you to start letting go.

Tip 5: Exercising

Exercise is an incredible way to release stress you are holding onto. When you exercise, your body releases chemicals called endorphins which trigger positive feelings in your body. Regular exercise can be a fantastic way to handle emotions because movement helps you to maintain emotional equilibrium.

There are countless ways you can exercise. You can go to a gym, go running, try high intensity interval training (HIIT), do strength training or any form of cardiovascular exercise. You could also do pilates, yoga, tai chi, or qigong. You can incorporate hiking, biking, paddleboarding or climbing into your life to increase your movement. Living a healthy lifestyle should incorporate a variety of these modalities. The main thing is to get your body moving, to get the blood circulating so that you can benefit from the feel-good endorphins. The endorphins increase your positive emotions and improve your mindset and this helps in healing.

Tip 6: Forgiveness

This is a big one. Forgiving others is an awesome way to free yourself from the past. Practicing forgiveness starts healing the feelings of hurt or betrayal you might feel towards certain people or past situations. Forgiveness is something you do for yourself. You forgive the other person to allow yourself to heal the hurt they caused you. Forgiving another does not mean that you are saying that what they did was okay. It is simply a way of releasing yourself in order to regain your inner peace.

While practicing forgiveness, it is important to forgive yourself as well. Very often, we are our own worst critics. We can be incredibly harsh towards ourselves. We might go over past events and think how we could have done something different or said something else. We can do this when it comes to thinking about our health as well and this can stop us from taking action to change the situation.

I used to be harshly critical of myself for not taking care of my body and that was very detrimental to me, because the emotions stopped me from doing anything about it. Once I forgave myself for how I had treated myself, I was able to move forward and make the changes I needed to make.

Self-forgiveness helps resolve any guilt, self-doubt and shame that we may have from past wrongdoings, incidents and traumas. We are then able to release the emotions associated with these events.

FINAL WORDS

Learning to love ourselves is difficult but it is worth it. When we love ourselves, we are accepting ourselves unconditionally and we have more self-confidence and self-worth. This helps us to support our physical, psychological and spiritual growth.

The tips I have included are all ways to practice self love. Start by doing something, take a small step. Begin today. That will help you to get started on your healing journey.

I am many steps forward now, releasing emotions I have been holding onto, learning to let go of things, confronting things. I am by far not done, as the layers come off and other things reveal themselves. But as I learn and as I make use of the above tools, it is starting to become easier little by little. Learning about my emotions has helped me to change my life and it is my wish that you, too, will learn about your emotions so that you can find your healthiest self.

The secret of health for both mind and body is not to mourn for the past, not to worry about the future, or not to anticipate troubles, but to live in the present moment wisely and earnestly.

~ BUDDHA

ABOUT THE AUTHOR

Priti is a life coach who, through her own experience, supports and helps people find their potential and direction of life through their inner guidance. Her vision is to empower people with tools which can be implemented easily into their daily lives, which in turn will help them grow in all areas of their lives by bringing in sustainable lifelong changes leading to a happy and healthy life transformation. She does this work using several modalities like NLP Practitioner, Time Line Therapy, Hypnotherapy and Holobody. She is also a lifelong student, always looking for alternative ways of healing, learning more about different ways of connecting with her higher self and spirituality.

Contact Information:
Email: priti8975@gmail.com
Instagram: @priti8975
LinkedIn: Priti Shah

PART 2
LIFESTYLE CHOICES: PHYSICAL HEALTH

Keeping your body healthy is an
expression of gratitude
to the whole cosmos-the trees,
the clouds, everything.

~THICH NHAT HANH

PART 2: PHYSICAL HEALTH

Our body is the only home we will live in. We must take care of our physical self in order to have the strength and energy to live the life we dream of living. In many cases though, we do not even know how to take care of our body. We grow up with a set of beliefs about how we should eat, drink and whether or not we should exercise. These beliefs come from our families and friends as well as the society that we are raised in.

The beliefs we hold around health are ingrained in us at such an early age that we don't even question them. We continue to eat the foods we are used to eating and to live the lifestyle we were trained to live. Whether this way of living is healthy is not even considered in many cases.

Many people become adults without having any real understanding of how they should treat their bodies. This lack of knowledge can result in weight gain and illness as the person gets older. Not knowing why they are gaining weight or getting sick means that the person makes no change and the situation continues to get worse.

This is the reason that having a solid understanding of health is essential to living a holistic lifestyle.

In this section, you will read truly transformational stories of people who overcame truly difficult and painful health situations. They are the stories of people who decided to take responsibility for their own physical health. Each person found a way to create a system of well-being that enabled them to reclaim their lives. The stories are powerful, as are the tools and techniques used by each person.

Remember, each person is different and each body is unique. There is no one-size-fits all answer to how to be in peak health. The tools and techniques in this section will give you an idea for a direction that may work for you. Ultimately, though, you must experiment and find the perfect combination of exercises and habits that work for you.

In this section you will find inspiring stories from people who found themselves in challenging health situations. These are the stories of their own personal dark night of the soul when they had to face the truth that they either had to change or they would continue down the path towards illness and disease. These are intimate stories about the way they faced their own personal difficulties, took responsibility and then went on their own personal journey towards ultimate health and wellness.

These stories are meant to inspire you to be brave, to face the truth, to take responsibility and then to take the journey. We will be walking right alongside you.

And I said to my body softly, 'I
want to be your friend.'
It took a long breath and replied, 'I have been
waiting my whole life for this.'

~*Nayyirah Waheed*

**How you love yourself is how you
teach others to love you.**

~Rupi Kaur

CHAPTER 9
A LOVE STORY
by Bruno Anjos

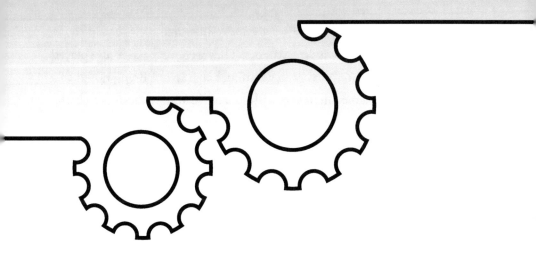

TOPIC:	Physical Health & Fitness
TOOL:	The Seven Lifestyle Needs
TECHNIQUE:	Assess yourself in each of the seven lifestyle needs and create a healthy plan of action for each area. The seven lifestyle habits are nutrient richness, frequent movement, sound sleep, inner stillness, deep connections, syncing with nature and a sense of purpose.

Wellness is the complete integration of body, mind and spirit—the realization that everything we do, think, feel and believe has an effect on our state of well-being.

~GREG ANDERSON

Well, I am a cancer zodiac, how could this be anything but a love story? And like every good love story, it has love and hate, it has happiness and sadness, it has excitement and anger. Love, like change, is incredible in the beginning, complicated and messy in the middle, but it can turn out to be quite amazing and totally worth it at that end, can't it?

This is the love story between me and my body. A long and complicated love story filled with highs and lows. Yes, we have a very healthy and loving relationship today, but it wasn't always like that.

I guess it all started with my parents. They were very active and played a lot of sports. My mom was even a national champion! Being raised in a sporty family made me fall in love with sports too and, without even being fully conscious of how it happened, I developed an early physical literacy. It was amazing. I could run, jump, catch, throw and kick. I could play literally any sport without needing much practice!

Credit also to my amazing body that, in the correct environment, was able to develop and express itself so brilliantly. At this point, I made a friend! A friend with whom I could play, a friend with whom I was having fun and, because of it and with it, I was exploring and discovering the world! My body was at its peak and I loved pushing the limits of what it could do.

Pretty early in my life, a new passion came, kicking a ball became my lifestyle, football became my love! It's all I cared about, the only thing I wanted to do.

Well, you all know what happens when you fall in love, don't you? You don't think about anyone or anything else besides your passion! And so, my amazing body, such a fantastic friend for so many years, the one I was discovering the world with, that I was playing with, was put aside, ignored. I didn't care how I treated it. In my relentless pursuit of my passion, my sport, I completely stopped taking care of my body.

Instead of making this a love triangle, me-body-football (anything is possible, why not?), I was selfishly using it while disregarding it. It's not that I was not providing it what it needed, at least the bare minimum, but it was not out of love, it was simply a means to an end; becoming a professional football player! I took my body for granted during these years.

There were times that I even blamed my body for my injuries. I would get frustrated when I got hurt and impatient with the time it took to heal. I often didn't even let my body fully heal before I was back to my sport. I pushed on regardless of how my body felt. Instead of taking care of my body, I pushed it beyond the limits as I focused on becoming a great football player.

As I grew older, I realized that I wasn't going to be able to fulfill my dream of becoming a professional footballer. My passion for football began to wane and I knew it was time to move on. Although my love for football never went away, I turned my attention towards my next chapter. University!

And thus it began. For those of you who were university students I'm sure you understand what happened then: endless parties, alcohol and smoking, long or sleepless nights of studying, a very rudimentary and unhealthy diet of tuna, pasta and tomato sauce. It was a time period where I was cold and disconnected from my body.

The way I was treating my body is actually very ironic because during university, I studied sports science. During this period, I gained unbelievable knowledge about the human body. I learned how it works and how it performs in different sports and activities. Yet even though I was learning this information and I was very active physically, I was still pushing and demanding things from my body and giving it practically nothing in return! What a friend Bruno, huh?!?

My mind and my heart were there, fully there, but I only called on my body when I needed it and normally pushed it too far beyond what was reasonable while my soul was pulling all the strings, trying to keep it all together.

Not long after finishing University, I decided to travel to China. First I was in Suiyang and then Shanghai and, as you might tell from a Portuguese born person, it was quite a shift in my life! My life wasn't as extreme as in my previous chapter but, even though I obviously brought my body with me, I didn't actually bring it. Do you know what I mean?

You see I had an average diet but I was regularly eating processed foods which were not nourishing me at all. On the weekends, I was abusing alcohol and staying out late. I had an irregular sleep schedule and although I never had trouble sleeping, I often felt tired. I ignored that. I kept being active, going to the gym and playing football over the weekends, but I followed the physical activity with abusive partying. Not exactly the best way to recover!

As far as stress was concerned, I thought I had a good relationship with stress because I always felt that stress pulls me to action. I even believed that being in stressful situations like being put on the spot or finishing work on deadlines was good for me, I felt it motivated me. Looking back, though, I really didn't have any healthy mechanisms for coping with stress. I would either close myself down or burst out and explode in anger when the pressure got too high. I'm guessing at least some of you can relate, right?

And then, Covid hit. Spring of 2020, who can forget! I was on a vacation in Indonesia, which was so lovely, when I first heard about Covid. When I returned to Shanghai, I returned to the first lockdown. I was alone, quarantined at home, in a country thousands of miles and several time zones away from home, from family and from friends. It hit me hard.

This was when my stress skyrocketed and since I had no coping mechanisms, many negative emotions started emerging on a regular basis. I was so grateful for technology during this time because online social connection and relationships were my oasis during these dark times. Remember, as I mentioned earlier, my birth sign is cancer. Like most cancers, I am very loving but when I fall, I fall hard. I have a tendency of being quite dramatic and can sometimes fall into depression.

It was such a strange time for me because although I was physically living in China, my heart, mind and soul was living in Portugal. I was living in China but I kept to the time zone of Portugal so I could stay in touch with my social network, my loved ones. I was waking up very late and going to bed very early the next day. I was binge-watching television, watching all the series and I was attacking all the snacks and alcohol bottles.

It was frightening because I felt like I was spiraling into a wormhole towards the darkness. I can only imagine, looking at the situation from an outside perspective, how my body could have felt, I mean it was living that same situation: it couldn't go out and enjoy the sunlight, it couldn't workout because I wasn't giving that to it, it wasn't resting well because of stress and messed up schedules, it wasn't eating well because of my choices and it wasn't feeling connection, not even from the soul it was carrying all along! I don't even know how it could handle all that without succumbing into the darkness towards which I was heading. As an amazing friend, it stayed there, it stayed put, it stayed strong throughout the difficult situation I was living in.

At this moment and as in every love story, you're expecting a big argument, a huge breakthrough and a gigantic and loving peace-making act. I hate to disappoint you but that was not what happened. This is not that "typical" love story.

You see, my body stayed strong, unbelievably hanging on without any motive, it patiently stood there waiting for me to be ready for a change, connecting with the universe to send me the right signals that would spark a change. Who would have thought that such a thing would happen?

During my endless and mindless sessions of binge-watching videos, I started to get some personal development advertisements, which I initially ignored. As time passed, I figured I had nothing to lose and I became curious. I decided to start watching personal development videos and my personal development journey began. It has remained a part of my life ever since and I am determined that it will be part of my daily life forever.

Stars were really aligning and I decided to take a health certification course. I learned all aspects of coaching including health, fitness, how to heal the body, how to tune into the body, lifestyle concerns and exercise. I wasn't just learning about these things. For once, I was also applying them to my own life and I was so happy that I was finally on the right path. That I was finally taking care of my body. I began to feel amazing in all ways. My body, mind and spirit were finally in alignment. I was finally on a healing journey of health and wellness.

Looking back upon my journey, one of the key things I realized was that I wasn't taking care of myself physically because I had never learned how to take care of it. I also realized that I had never learned to truly love my body, to truly love myself. I was able to love other people but not myself.

Throughout this whole process of personal development and growth, one thing that I really learned was self-love and self-care. I learned to love all things about myself. I discovered that I am perfectly imperfect and that, oh that, was a priceless gift that made me look at myself in a different way.

I began to see everything differently. Instead of looking at the outcome, being focused on the goal, I was looking at the process. I was celebrating my progress and not my results. I was learning how to best take care of my body by examining what I was eating and drinking. I looked at how much exercise I was getting and whether that was beneficial exercise for me personally. I learned to control myself by feeling grateful to my body and moving into a state where I wanted to take care of it. I also released a lot of negative behaviors and emotions and simply let the rest be. I let the universe and my guardians take care of it. In the end, they will always have my back and will give me what I need to evolve.

The big redemption piece of this love, of my reconciliation with my body, is a practice that I learned through my certification course called "Body talk". It's incredible the way I was evolving and growing but still disregarding my body. My body was the only thing that allowed me to live in this world. My body, which was my first and most loyal friend.

I had a lot of apologizing to do to my body, I had to make amends, I had to recognize all those years that I had selfishly used it without acknowledgment, I had to make up for all the times I pushed way beyond its limits and, even then, it always stayed strong, loyal, by my side, loving me and providing me the amazing life experience I had been having.

It is a very beautiful and liberating process to get to know your body, to talk to your body. It's just you and your body. You can write to it, you can talk to it. You can stand in front of the mirror and truly look at your body and feel gratitude for the truly magnificent machine that it is. It's strange and a little uncomfortable in the beginning, but as soon as you connect, it's an indescribable experience. You can really go deep and feel your body communicating with you.

It was an intense experience for me. I understood how I had treated my body and for the first time, I poured all my heart out and fully apologized to my body. I also made a commitment to my body. I promised that I would always appreciate and acknowledge my body. I would love my body and develop a symbiotic and harmonious life with it. This commitment has allowed me to express my maximum potential and fully experience the world!

Yeah, like you are probably thinking, my body said "finally!" and I felt this loving energy throughout my whole being. I also promised my body and myself, that I will make it my mission to leave nobody behind! No body behind! I decided I would teach everyone I could the body talk exercise. These conversations can be very powerful, believe me and they can change the whole direction of your health, body and lifestyle.

Once I did the body talk exercise, I knew what I needed to do. I needed to cherish my body and to take care of it. I learned about the seven lifestyle needs and I decided to create a healthy lifestyle around this unique format that I learned in my Holobody certification.

THE SEVEN LIFESTYLE NEEDS

The seven lifestyle needs are nutrient richness, frequent movement, sound sleep, inner stillness, deep connections, syncing with nature and a sense of purpose.

Assessment:

Here's how you do it

1. *Inventory:* First, do an inventory in each of these categories, without changing anything. Be honest about where you actually are in each area and dive deep as you gain a true understanding and awareness about your habits.

2. *Beliefs:* Next, examine your beliefs around each of the seven lifestyle needs. Question each of your beliefs and feel free to let go of the ones that are not working for you. This process can be quite eye-opening because sometimes we have beliefs ingrained in us from a very young age that were not even created by us, we just unconsciously inherited them. Removing these blocks is essential.

3. *Vision:* The next step is to define your vision. Determine where you want to go and define what your perfect state or situation within each area would be. This vision should be very clear.

4. *Your Why:* Once you have your vision, determine your why. Why do you want to achieve this vision in each of the seven areas of health? You might discover your why during your body talk exercise. Discover a powerful reason for living at peak health and fitness. This is your reason, your why.

5. *Create Your Plan:* Finally, you must make a plan. Define the steps you need to take to achieve your vision, What steps make sense for you and your purpose? What steps will bring you closer to your ideal self?

Habits and Routines:

I believe that we all have massive potential. Our potential is truly huge and limitless. In order to move towards the grandest version of ourselves, it is imperative to have habits and routines that enhance your ability to fully express your potential. Here are some of the practices I have incorporated into my life. They have worked for me and I invite you to try them to see which ones will work for you.

Sleep:

Have you ever realized that after a poor night of sleep you feel terrible? Sleep affects our emotions and it clouds our judgment. It can lead to negative thinking patterns and unhealthy thoughts. Not getting enough sleep can lead to cravings and unhealthy desires.

In order to truly perform at the top of your game, you must optimize your sleep. Focus on keeping a regular sleep schedule, going to sleep and waking up at the same time each day. If possible, link your sleep to the rhythm of nature by going to sleep when it is dark and getting up when the sun is rising. This allows you to align your circadian rhythm.

Here is a very catchy sleep rule: the 8-4-3-2-1-0 rule. Stop drinking any type of caffeine eight hours before bed; stop intense exercise four hours before sleep; stop eating three hours before bed; stop working and drinking two hours before bed; stop using technology and electronic devices one hour before sleep; and hit the snooze button zero times in the morning.

What can make everything even easier? Controlling the environment where you sleep. Your bed should be used for love or for sleep only. Training yourself in this manner signals to your brain that getting into bed means it is time to relax. Make sure that your bedroom is clutter free and make it as dark as possible, even adding room darkening shades to get the best night rest you can.

Stress:

Stress relieving techniques are essential to a healthy life. Practices for handling stress are essential to promote inner peace, harmony and to maintain a sense of presence and groundedness.

Meditation is a great way to manage stress. There are so many benefits to meditation but the traditional way we think about meditation is that we should totally clear our mind and sit totally thought free. This is passive meditation and it can be difficult for many of us.

There is another option, however. There is a type of meditation called active meditation and this is a guided meditation. Guided meditations can be found online via many websites and apps, but you can also create your own guided meditation by recording one on your phone and using that to meditate.

While meditating, you can focus on a topic like love, compassion, gratitude, or forgiveness. When meditating on love, make a list of all the people, places and things that you love. A compassion meditation would be where you seek to feel compassion for all people, animals, plants and insects. Alternatively, you could meditate on gratitude and feel grateful for all the amazing things in your life.

Nutrition:

A great way to approach nutrition is by using a combination of whole foods, and increased protein intake. These all work together synergistically to create a healthy approach to diet.

The best way to eat is to focus on whole foods, which are natural and more nutritious. These whole foods contain everything needed to nourish the body as they are dense in vitamins and minerals. Aim to avoid the dangers and toxicity of processed foods as they contain lots of unnecessary and unhealthy added ingredients that are used to keep the processed food fresh. These added ingredients are often toxic to the body.

It is important to make sure that you have adequate protein intake each day. Protein is an absolutely essential macronutrient which is necessary for everyone. There is a common misconception that only bodybuilders need protein, but the truth is that we all need protein.

If you focus on these areas, you won't even have to worry about calorie tracking or strict diets. Diet culture has created a lot of unhealthy behaviors because typically diets are highly restrictive and not easy to maintain. By shifting the focus to healthy eating and approaching nutrition as a way to nourish your body and to make it strong, you will find that it is easy to make the right choices. And don't forget, if you notice you are making some poor food choices, go back to your body talk and find out why you are eating as you are.

Physical Activity:

Having an active lifestyle is key to living a long, healthy life. It is essential to keep your body strong but also supple and flexible. Find an exercise routine that works for you, one that you will stick to. It is important to pair exercise with fun, active hobbies like walking, running, or hiking. Spending time outdoors as you engage in these activities will enhance your well-being even more.

FINAL WORDS

It is my hope that my story will be valuable to you. I hope it inspires you and helps you to go on your own health journey. Please remember that each of us are different, so the ideas in this chapter are a starting point for you. Try them and see what works for you. Once you incorporate those things into your life, experiment with other ways you can add health and fitness into your life. Make it a lifestyle.

Remember, you are much more than simply your body, but your body is your only and unreplaceable vehicle to live and experience this world, treat it well and your life will become limitless! Love your body, love yourself!

Physical fitness is the first requisite of happiness.
~JOSEPH PILATES

ABOUT THE AUTHOR

Bruno Anjos is a Portuguese and World Citizen in love with people and the abundance and infinite possibilities of human achievement and potential!

Bruno holds a Master in Sports Science. He is a Football (Soccer) Coach, a Physical & Health Education Teacher, Health Education Coordinator and a Holistic Health, Fitness & Lifestyle Coach. He holds coaching certifications in Holobody and 10X.

He is a growth seeker and an everlasting learner. His mission is to raise the consciousness that humans only live in this world given that they have a body that allows their presence and their experience. Bruno's mission is to leave no body behind by making sure that his clients have a fully expressed health and body. He coaches his clients in all aspects of health so that they have all the conditions necessary for them to achieve their true and ultimate potential!

Contact Information:
Author's Socials
WhatsApp/Telegram - +351914152357
LinkedIn: https://www.linkedin.com/in/coachbrunoanjos/
WeChat - CoachBrunoAnjos
Email - anjox123@hotmail.com
Facebook - https://www.facebook.com/brunomrdosanjos
Website/Facebook Page - https://www.facebook.com/coachbrunoanjos/
Instagram - https://www.instagram.com/coachbrunoanjos/

**Motivation is what gets you started.
Habit is what keeps you going.**

~Jim Rohn

The successful person makes a habit of doing what the failing person doesn't like to do.

~Thomas Edison

CHAPTER 10

SAFETY NET ROUTINE: YOUR LIFELINE

by Kim Stumne

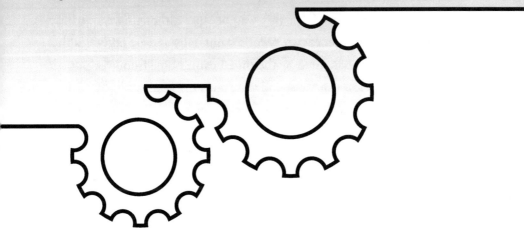

TOPIC: Creating Sustainable Habits

TOOL: Safety Net Routines

TECHNIQUE: Create a goal and then make a minimum safety net routine which is a routine that you can fall back on even when you don't have enough time. Use the safety net routine to install new habits and to maintain them.

The body loves routine.
Try to eat, sleep and so on at the same times every day
in order for the body to function at its optimum
efficiency. The body loves consistency.

~THERESA HEARN HAYNES

Are you waiting for the perfect time to implement new health habits or for the next new "magic pill" to come out that will make you a healthier version of you? Don't hold your breath.

This is exactly where I was a few years ago, I kept waiting for the perfect time to start and I was looking for short cuts that would improve my health. They never came.

I was tired, overwhelmed, distracted and had no time to focus on my health. I wasn't sure why I felt this way because although I was a busy professional and a mother of two, I worked out daily and ate fairly healthy. However, I was still exhausted by the time I came home from work. It felt like I had less and less time to spend time with my family.

Then, when I turned 37, I noticed that I had started to have less energy than ever before. I had lost my passion to create a fantastic life and it truly felt like I was living on autopilot.

Have you ever felt like you were watching your life like it was a movie? LIke you were just going through the motions, not really participating? Have you ever felt like it wasn't even your life you were leading? This is what I felt like. It was the feeling that I was not showing up or fulfilling my life's purpose. I felt beaten down physically, emotionally, mentally and spiritually. I wondered, is this what life is all about?

One day at a doctor's appointment I complained to my doctor about having fatigue, feeling bloated, having brain fog and needing more caffeine to get me through the day. I asked her what I could do to fix this. She looked at me, chuckled and said, "You're getting older, you have two kids, you work 50-hour work weeks and you're finishing your master's degree. You should be tired. It is just part of getting older."

I went home and thought about what my doctor had said. This one statement swirled around my head for days and weeks. I wasn't sure what to make of it. I swayed back and forth between "Yes she's probably right and I just have to accept this" to "Why does it have to be this way?"

I began to journal and put down all the thoughts I was having. I was arguing back and forth with myself as I grappled with the issue of my health.

The journaling led me to realize that I was not willing to accept what my doctor had said. I was committing to do something else. That was when I made the decision to go on a transformational journey to find another way.

It wasn't easy to go against what my doctor said. It wasn't only my doctor, either. Everywhere I turned, the message was the same. Health and wellness declined as you got older. This was normal. Everybody accepted this message.

But I was not going to accept what the world told me was "normal" and I wanted to find a way to optimize my health in the most efficient way possible. I chose to create a life and a body that would support the experiences I wanted to have in the time that I lived on this earth. I made a commitment to myself that I would find another way. That I would find a way to live a life where I was healthy and happy.

When did it become ok for others to dictate how we should feel, look, or the life we live? This one question sent me on a journey of discovery and health transformation. I discovered many tools, tips and techniques that helped me to regain the same level of health and fitness that I had as a young woman.

This journey has been filled with so many amazing moments. It hasn't always been easy, but I am proud that I stuck with it. I am so proud of myself that I have come so far and now, here I am, three years later. My life is completely different. I am healthy and I feel motivated and excited about life. I am in a place now that instead of watching a movie I have no control over, I am rewriting my script every day to be the best version of me.

I studied many different health modalities and learned a lot of techniques to improve my health. One of the best tools I have found is called the Safety Net Routine. It is a true gamechanger. It has worked wonders for me and the best thing is that it is a routine that is easy to learn and easy to execute.

Do you want more energy, a body that can keep up with your life's aspirations and the ability to create new habits that are aligned with where you want to be? The answer is simple: start using the tool safety net routines today. This easy to implement tool will help you to transform your life, your health and your work, by aligning new habits with the experiences you want to create in your life.

THE SAFETY NET ROUTINE: YOUR LIFELINE

Safety Net Routines are the minimum version of a habit you want in your life. The safety net routine streamlines your healthy habits into a doable routine, one that will lay the groundwork for healthy living. By implementing a safety net routine, you are establishing the habit in such a way that you consider yourself to be a success.

An example of this would be if your health goal was to go to the gym three times a week and work out for 20 minutes each time, your safety net routine could be to do a 5-minute workout at the gym.

You may be thinking, how will a five-minute workout help me transform my health? Well, it isn't meant to totally transform your health. Instead, a safety net routine is meant to help you shift your mindset and keep you motivated to stick with your new habit.

Have you ever had a setback that completely knocked out your motivation? Or started a new diet and then gave up when you ate a piece of cake or junk food? Maybe you began an exercise routine and then missed going to the gym for a few days in a row and then never went back. This happens to everyone. We set a goal and then when we don't achieve it or when we stumble and fall, we give up completely.

Think about why this happens. When you fail to meet your goal, how did it make you feel about your will power to continue the new healthy habits? If you are anything like me, you felt like a failure and thought that maybe you would never be able to improve your health. It might make you lose your trust in yourself and give up your belief that you could successfully create any long-term change or transformation.

Worse yet these stumbles make us feel depleted. Our energy seems to spiral down.

This can lead to a loss of motivation. This is when we drop into procrastination behavior and before you know it, you are back into your old habits. You turn away from the promises you made to yourself about the new healthy habits and you go back to your old ways of living.

This is why safety net routines can be your saving grace. They can be your lifeline to the change you desire. When you learn new habits, you need to do more than just replace the bad habit with a good one. You need to teach your brain to change in order to support the new habit. By installing a minimum basic safety net routine, you will be more likely to maintain it and this success will help to support the new habit. Eventually the new habit results in a permanent shift in your behavior.

Creating safety net routines for every new habit allows the brain to get familiar with the new habit. Once your brain repeats the habit over and over, it triggers a muscle memory response which allows the new habit to be automatic. It's like you are on autopilot because the new habit has become second nature.

Instilling the basic minimum new habit gives the person a trigger to celebrate their success and this further solidifies the new habit by keeping motivation high. Suddenly the insurmountable goals become easier and you start to give gratitude for the goals you have already achieved.

HEALTH TRANSFORMATION

The journey to a health transformation focuses on seven human needs: nutrient richness, frequent movement, sound sleep, inner stillness, deep connection, being in sync with nature and a sense of purpose.

Starting with the need that has the most impact on my concerns of fatigue and lack of energy helped me to slowly build habits that were sustainable instead of changing habits that fit in all seven categories at once. The starting point for me was sound sleep, creating a new evening routine to wind down. I made sure to create a great evening routine. I made sure that I had my last meal at least two hours before my bedtime, I ensured

I had no blue light for one hour prior to bed and I did at least five minutes of meditation directly before I went to sleep. Adding these behaviors drastically changed the quality and quantity of my sleep, which in turn boosted my energy levels.

Using the safety net routine concept helped me to establish this routine and even on nights where I am pressed for time, I am able to institute this basic routine. The safety net routine I created for my evening routine was to have no blue light for five minutes before bed, ending my meal at least one hour before bed and meditating by paying attention as I took ten deep breaths with my eyes closed. Each day that I was able to do my safety net routine I celebrated it as a win and congratulated myself. This kept me motivated and as time went by, implementing my evening routine seemed easier and easier as the days passed.

As I began to create this evening routine, I wondered why it is that we can be more successful in creating a new habit if we focus on one to two things at a time? Fun fact, the brain takes on 11,000,000 bits of information, but can only process 40 bits of information at one time. This means that we need to do things in small pieces in order to be successful.

Oftentimes, when people want to transform their lives or health, they implement every new habit they can think of at the same time and then wonder why they are not successful. The key is to start with small, buildable habits by creating safety net routines. Starting small like this will improve your chances of success. Sticking to this non-negotiable safety net routine can improve all areas of your life: your work, your health, your fitness, your well-being, your sleep and your motivation in the early stages of habit building. Having a tool like safety net routines helps you to uplevel your life in order to get to the next level.

As you begin your journey towards ultimate health and well-being, try the safety net routine technique. Start by making a goal and then also create a minimum safety net that will satisfy you and make you feel like you are succeeding. You will be amazed at how easily you bring new healthy habits into your life.

REAL TALK

Will safety net routines be your one and only tool you need to change your health, fitness, or life; or will this suddenly make all change easy? The answer is no, there is not one tool that will work like a miracle pill, believe me, I have tried everything. However, these routines are a critical tool that help you create sustainability and continued action towards your goals. This is what creates transformation.

This tool will shift your mindset positively, instead of feeling like a failure every time you have a day where you don't meet your main goal. These safety net routines keep you motivated, supporting you and keeping you on the right track. They give you the grace and compassion for yourself that you need to succeed. They remind you that you do not have to be perfect. Imperfect action is still action and it helps to propel you forward to achieve your goals. It also empowers you to take a deep dive into what you really want for your health. Begin to learn about different health techniques and you will eventually discover what you want for your health and what experiences you want to have in life.

Looking back at what I have accomplished, I want to share with you how much has changed for me by using these safety net routines. I have shifted from a reactive health state where I was treating symptoms once they arose to a proactive health state where I focus on adding various practices to my life that keep my body healthy. I love to research and then experiment with what my body needs. I create new habits that are sustainable using safety net routines.

Up until a year ago, I would have never imagined that my life, body and mindset would be where it is today. I started to listen to what my body was saying it needed versus taking on someone else's version of what to expect from my health. Using safety net routines, I had my own health transformation. I created new sustainable habits that allowed me to reduce my caffeine intake, improve my sleep and take the time to connect with myself through journaling and meditation. I created a morning and evening routine, added micro workouts daily and started resistance training twice a week, which drastically improved my muscle quality and metabolic health. These habits allowed me to have more energy than ever before and more time to have the experiences that bring me joy.

Change does not need to be complicated, if all you have is five minutes then use those five minutes wisely. It is about buildable habits, the old idea that you need to make massive habit changes to see massive transformations no longer holds true. It is the small, consistent changes you do that create a ripple effect that can transform your health and life.

Are you ready to stop living in the "status quo" and decide what health looks like for you? If so, start today. Begin with one tiny new habit and build from there. In a year, you will be amazed at what you have achieved.

KEY TAKEAWAYS

- Start with small, buildable habits
- Focus on one or two health needs at a time
- Use this list to decide what area you want to focus on first.
  - Nutrient richness
  - Frequent movement
  - Sound sleep
  - Inner stillness
  - Deep connection
  - Being in sync with nature
  - A sense of purpose

QUESTIONS TO ASK YOURSELF

- Why is this goal important to you?
- How will achieving this goal positively impact your health?
- What new habit do you want to create to help you fulfill this health need?

- What is the non-negotiable minimal routine that you would deem as a success? This is your safety net routine for this new goal.
- How will you celebrate your successes?

Review this list when you are trying to make any changes, or creating new habits that seem difficult to change. Remember that change takes time. Think about how many times you fell and had to get back up when you first learned to ride a bike. Implementing any new habit is the same. It takes persistence and practice. Keep at it. No matter how many times you fall or feel like you fail, get back up. Change will happen if you keep trying.

We are not born with the innate ability to change at the drop of a hat and many of our habits are created from years of beliefs and experiences that supported the habits we have now. It makes sense that it will take time to create new beliefs and habits to support those new beliefs. Be patient with yourself throughout this process.

I have come to realize that my health is no longer a destination to get to, but a journey that is ever evolving. Remember that we are all on a journey of growth and it is the journey that matters. We are creating our lives much like an artist creates a work of art. Seeing your life through this lens allows you to see the beauty in every success and every "failure", the experiences we have shape the person we are and who we will become. I know that my health journey will never be perfect and that is ok. I do know that the journey will always be mine.

I hope my story has inspired you to get ready to take imperfect action towards your goals so that your body can become the beautiful work of art it truly is.

With love,
Kim

ABOUT THE AUTHOR

Kim Stumne is a wife, mother, nurse leader and coach. She has spent years finding ways to optimize her own health, fitness and wellness, but this did not come easily. She is here to share her failures, research and success with you to allow you to achieve your own personal health goals.

Contact Info:
Website- www.empoweredhealthllc.coach
Instagram- https://www.instagram.com/kim_rn_coach/
LinkedIn- www.linkedin.com/in/kim-stumne-562008166
Link Tree: https://linktr.ee/kim_rn_coach

We are all a work of art.

~Ajit Nawalkha

**A journey of a thousand miles
begins with one step.**

~Lao Tzu

CHAPTER 11

RUNNING: MY ACTIVE MEDITATION

by Patrick Morrison

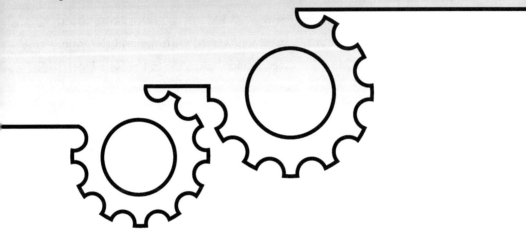

TOPIC:	Cardiovascular Fitness
TOOL:	Running
TECHNIQUE:	Add a great cardiovascular workout like running into your life.

It is a rough road that leads to the heights of greatness.

~ SENECA

My journey began with my son. In 2020. He did a book report for a school assignment where he created a top ten style video. I was very proud and impressed with what he came up with all on his own.

I decided to take a page out of his book and make my own video. As we all know, 2020 was a tough year, but I decided to make a video to highlight everything we had to celebrate in 2020, because not everything was bad. When I told my son that he had inspired me to make a video of the best things in 2020, his comment was "What are you celebrating? Beer?"

I chuckled at first, but his statement stayed with me and the more I thought about it, the more I realized it had shaken me to the core. I started to question many of my life choices. Was this really the message I wanted to give my young impressionable son? Did I want him to grow up thinking that his dad needed alcohol to have a good time? How could I be a better example and role model to this young person? What memories did I want him to have of me when he grew up? His comment was the main trigger for my desire to change. It was the impetus I needed to realize that I wanted to be a better husband to my wife and a better father to my children.

Now, before I get into my journey and where it has taken me, I must first explain where I came from. I started drinking when I was 13, which is the age my son is now and I started doing drugs shortly thereafter. I was running away from reality and from responsibility. I was trying to hide my feelings of inadequacy.

Like many teenagers, I was trying to fit in and my behaviors were fueled by my constant need to be liked and to please others. I did not feel that I was able to be my true self for fear of being judged or ridiculed. I had preconceived notions on how men should act in society and I struggled to fit into the mold.

I carried many of these insecurities, as well as the need to fit in and to please others, through my teenage years and well into adulthood. My visions of what a man should be and what manhood meant dictated how I acted. I wanted to be accepted so I conformed to what I was taught about masculinity. As humans, we are tribal beings and the need to fit in is ingrained in our DNA. Historically, to be kicked out of a tribe meant certain death.

However, this constant need to belong and to fit in no longer serves us well today. It certainly wasn't serving me well.

In 2020, when the world shut down, I went deeper and deeper into drinking and chasing what I thought was a good time. But when my son, who was himself getting to the age I was when it all began for me, teased me about the beer, it flicked a switch in me. I knew there was more to life than what I was doing. I knew that I had a bigger purpose and I knew that I needed to be a better example for him. I knew that the people closest to me deserved the best version of myself. I also knew that where I was and who I was, were due to a collection of my own choices and that by making new choices, I could change into someone I was proud of. I knew I was capable of so much more.

I had to learn to love myself and to treat my body better than what I had been doing. It was time for change and for self-reflection. It was time to start taking care of a body that I had neglected for a long time. I started to invest time, money and energy into bettering myself, physically, mentally and spiritually.

One thing I have learned on my journey is that self-care and self-love is not selfish. We cannot pour from an empty cup.

As I began to reflect upon my life, I thought about running. I did not start running in 2020 when I made the decision to turn my life around. In fact, I have been running for many years. I started running in 2005 with my first 10-kilometer race and slowly trained my way to my first marathon a couple years later.

Once I had hit the pinnacle of achievements for runners, I transitioned into triathlons, starting with a Try-Tri distance and again working my way up over several years to a full Ironman. An Ironman race consists of a 4-kilometer swim, a 180-kilometer bike and a 42.2-kilometer run.

I can tell you from experience that finishing a race such as this requires a lot of planning, training, dedication and support and that the feeling you get when the master of ceremonies announces that "Patrick, you are an Ironman," is like no other moment.

Yet despite all these achievements, ones that many will never be able to claim in their lives, I was still not happy with myself. I was still running away from who I was and what I could be. I never gave my training for these races my full dedication, as I was always afraid that it would not be enough. I feared that I would give my all and be disappointed with the results, so I made sure that I always had excuses and a safety net. While I was putting my body through the grueling training required for an Ironman race, I was still drinking on weekends. It was a paradox.

After much self-reflection, I can see now that it was a form of self-sabotage. I knew that if I somehow failed or got to the finish line with a result less than I had hoped, I would have an excuse ready. I could blame it on the fact that I had taken weekends off, or had not really given it my all, or had not really trained as hard as I could have. With every race I registered for, I told myself it would be different, but again and again I found myself falling into the same trap of finding ways to slow down my own progress.

MINDSET SHIFT

In 2020, when my journey truly began, I realized that my mindset had to be corrected. I realized that I was running and training as a punishment. I had been seeing it as the only way to maintain my unhealthy lifestyle. Running was a way to keep eating and drinking whatever I wanted. It was easy to justify eating unhealthy food or having a few drinks because I was very active and had run many kilometers that day or that week. But what if, instead of a punishment, running became a place of renewal, reflection and resilience? What if I could finally love my body and everything it has done for me? What if I started treating myself with the care and respect I deserved?

What if I could train and give my all to self-improvement without excuses and the need to create a safety net in case of failure? What if I started setting goals and working to achieve them instead of sabotaging myself? What if I could use my knowledge and background and everything that I have been through to inspire others to get moving and to show them that they, too, are capable of so much more? Many people are afraid to set impossible goals for fear of failure, but nothing is impossible. The word itself says "I'm possible". My "I'm possible" goal is to win my age group in the next triathlon race that I participate in.

For the first time, I believe in myself and I believe I can do it. That is the first step. The second step is to put in the work required to achieve it. My second goal and this one may be even more important, is to show you that you can achieve whatever "I'm possible" goal you set in your life.

If you are taking the time to read this, then you, like me, no longer want to fit in, or just get by. You want to become the best version of yourself. If you do not like the person who is staring back at you in the mirror, then maybe it's time for you to step up as well. You can choose to be the captain of your own ship. The journey of self-development is continuous, as the more you develop, the more you become self-aware and find new opportunities for growth and bettering yourself.

It can be difficult at the beginning, as it is easy to judge yourself when you slip off the path, but it is important to be gentle with yourself. Keep moving forward and strive every day to be just a little bit better than you were the day before. If you are just starting on your own journey and you are interested in getting healthy and adding some running to your routine (whether your goal is 5 kilometers, a marathon, or an Ironman), here are a few very important items that I would like you to consider. I will go into a bit more details on each one below:

Tips for Running

1. Preparation: Get a gait analysis and the correct shoes
2. Taking Action: Start out slowly, even if this just means walking a couple times a day and gradually build your body up to running.
3. Motivation: Sign up for a race even if it is just a local 5-kilometer race in your community
4. Accountability: Find a running group or running partner, or hire a coach

Tip 1: Preparation: Proper Running Shoes

The first item and probably the most important, is to get the proper shoes. Running shoes are the most important piece of equipment that you will own as a walker or runner. If possible, visit a local running specialty store and have your gait analyzed. Some stores will even do this virtually. The analysis will determine whether you pronate, supinate, or have a neutral gait and this will determine the correct pair of running shoes for you.

Tip 2: Taking Action: Start Out Slow

Once you have found the proper shoes, it is important to start out slowly, especially if you have never run before. This will allow your body to gradually adapt and can help avoid injury. For someone who is just starting out with running, I typically recommend a progressive schedule, such as the one below. This can be adapted if you are already athletic, or already do some running.

Starter Running Schedule

Step 1: Start with a walk around the block (10-15 minutes) 2 to 3 times a day. This should bring your daily steps in the range of 8,000 to 10,000 steps. Do this for 2 weeks.

Step 2: Once you have made daily walking a habit for a couple weeks, you can start incorporating some running. Run from one light post to the next, then walk to the third light post. Continue alternating between walking and running on your walk around the block. Do this for one of your daily walks 3 times a week (for example on Monday, Wednesday and Friday) for 2 weeks. You should also strive to maintain your daily walks on the days you are not running.

Step 3: Instead of running and walking between light posts, you will now add a timed interval to your runs. To start, you will run for 1 minute and then walk for 1 minute, alternating between running and walking. Do this three times a week for the first week. Once again, work to get your daily steps in on the days you are not running. Our bodies are meant to be moving and daily movement will keep the rust away.

Step 4: Finally, keep gradually increasing your running time by one minute per week while keeping your one-minute walking break. For example, on the second week, you would run for two minutes and walk for one minute, alternating between the two. This allows your body to adjust to slightly longer running times each week. A good goal to work towards would be to reach a point where you can comfortably run for 20 minutes without any walk breaks.

Tip 3: Motivation: Sign Up for a Race

The third item on my list is designed to help you get and keep the motivation to run. By signing up for a race, even a small one, you have an end goal in mind and something to work towards. For timing, keep in mind that the average runner can prepare for a 5-kilometer race in about 8 weeks, a 10-kilometer race in about 12 weeks, a half marathon (21.1 kilometers) in about 16 weeks and 18 weeks or more for a full marathon (42.2 kilometers).

Tip 4: Accountability: Find a Running Group or Partner

The final item on my list helps with your accountability. Joining a running group or finding a running partner will add a level of accountability to help avoid missing those runs on days where your personal motivation may be lower. Having a friend who is counting on you to show up will help keep you motivated. We all have days when we just do not feel like running, but those usually end up being the best runs when we force our body to move in that direction and we get it done.

For those very serious about taking up running, getting a coach is also a great alternative. A coach will provide you with a specific program, track your progress and help you reach the next level much faster than you would on your own.

FINAL WORDS

If I can leave you with one thought, it is that all things are possible if you believe that they are.

I am grateful that you have stayed with me this long. Perhaps you will be the next to decide that it is time to become the best version of yourself. All that is really needed is the will to become the leader of your own life and the decision to make it happen.

I would encourage you to ask yourself why you are here and what is your purpose. If you have not found it yet, I implore you to continue asking yourself the question until you do, because once you find out what lights you up, you will be unstoppable. For now, I will pass you the baton so that you may start setting and attaining your own "I'm possible" goals.

If you were inspired to begin a running practice by reading this chapter, please reach out to me, I would love to hear from you.

~Patrick

People with goals succeed because they know where they're going.

~ EARL NIGHTINGALE

ABOUT THE AUTHOR

Patrick Morrison was born and raised in Toronto, Canada. After hitting a crossroads in 2020 at the age of 41, he decided that he had more to give and began a journey of personal development. A Certified 10X Fitness & HoloBody coach by Evercoach Mindvalley.

Patrick is also an accomplished triathlete. When he is not swimming, biking, or running, he is inspiring and motivating our next generation of leaders.

His story is compelling and reminds us that it is never too late to start your journey.

Contact Info:
Linkedin: https://www.linkedin.com/in/patrick-morrison-3615908a/
Instagram: https://www.instagram.com/pmorr09/
Facebook: https://www.facebook.com/patrick.morrison.52090/
Facebook Group: https://www.facebook.com/groups/2716233501959982

He who has health, has hope and he who has hope, has everything.

~Thomas Carlyle

CHAPTER 12

MY FOREVER MEDICINE: 10X STRENGTH TRAINING

by Stéphanie Escorial

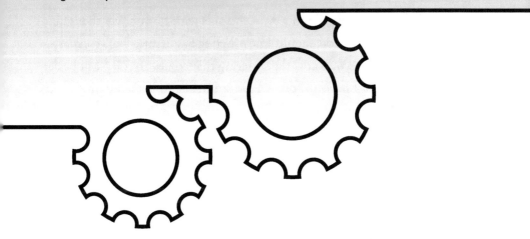

TOPIC:	Strength Training
TOOL:	10X Fitness Program
TECHNIQUE:	Two 15 minute strength workouts twice per week

*When the unthinkable happens, the lighthouse is hope.
Once we choose hope, everything is possible.*

~CHRISTOPHER REEVE

As I gather my accumulated pile of pills, I stun myself with how many there are. That's the way Dad did it, surely this will work. As I relish with determination to end the pain once and for all, a thought comes across, "You can't do this to Mum, you can't do this to your family."

I wake myself up from the inexplicable dark twisted energy, engulfing me with a distorted perception — there's no way out. "You must end it now."

I hear Mum next door and I drop the pills with horror. My thoughts turn to torment me, "You should know better Stéphanie, you've experienced the aftermath, you know the suffering that comes after it." I sit back and reflect on what I have just done. I am stunned and shaken to my core, on how close I came to death. Death was luring me and opening itself up to my suffering.

2008 was the point of no return, it was the beginning of a long journey to freeing myself from my own generational shackles.

It was a beautiful sunny afternoon in London and I had prepared a menswear collection for months. It was going to be fantastic and I was super excited. I had settled on a Futurist Abstract theme. I had carefully designed each piece. I had handpicked the luxurious fabrics from several stores in London and collaborated with a sought after menswear catwalk pattern cutter from the early 1990's to finalize the futuristic shapes. If David Bowie were alive today, it would be something right up his alley. I loved the collection.

I had organized six beautiful men to showcase my work and we were all excitedly making our way to the venue for the catwalk show.

As I sat at the back of the cab, I was excited. It was an excitement mixed with nervousness but mostly, I was eager to get to the venue, eager to see all my hard work come to life, showcased for the world to see.

All was going well until suddenly, I felt my body furiously jerking forward. The cab had hit another car. It awakened me from my illusionary trance to the present moment and I found myself in the midst of a confusing, destined event. I shook my head as I tried to make sense and construct some sort of order in my mind. The police were called and I started to panic about the show.

I frantically checked my body physically and nothing seemed out of place. I walked away without injury, or so I had thought and I grabbed another cab to get to the show without delay. I never stopped to actually process what just happened. I had to get to the show and nothing would stop me. My adrenaline carried me through and I continued onto the venue as if nothing had happened.

When I got to the venue, the preparations were underway. The excitement was palpable backstage as everyone buzzed around making it happen. Before I knew it, the music started and my dream materialized. I watched, transfixed as my creations were unveiled for the first time. I felt an incredible sense of accomplishment and joy.

It was an amazing night and the show was a success! I was flying high from the entire experience. The lights, the sound, the gorgeous men, my beautiful clothing. It was incredible and I felt like I was floating. My body felt light, almost as if I were invisible as the dopamine and serotonin flooded my system.

That night I decided to celebrate it big. We went out after the show and had a fabulous time. I let loose as I danced wildly, rejoicing in my win. Ah, what a night!

The next day I awakened with a banging headache. I figured it was all the fun of the after party. As I woke up, I released myself from my lover's soft embrace. As I moved out of the bed, I felt a potent ache in my neck. I wondered what that was from, but figured it was from all the dancing.

As the day progressed, my body began to ache more and more. I realized that this was a result of the cab accident, but I figured it would pass quickly. Unfortunately, that was not to be. As the days passed, my pain continued to progress until my lower back began to ache so badly that I found myself bedridden. I went to see a doctor who advised me to rest and allow myself to heal.

This began a three year period where my physical functioning was severely restricted. Those years were filled with pain, but I did everything I had to do. I spent those years after the accident going to endless sessions of physiotherapy, acupuncture, yoga classes and I added in strength training at the gym. A lot of my pain resolved, but I somehow couldn't shift my constant pins and needles on the soles of my feet.

Something was still not right.

I began developing a burning sensation inside my groin. I was misdiagnosed with vaginal atrophy and I was advised to apply lubricant and birth control patches to increase my estrogen level. The birth control patches were a big no for me, however occasionally I would apply the lubricant, but it didn't really help, so I learned to tolerate the discomfort for years.

I was physically unfit and I had gained 10 kg by my late thirties. The small tire around my hips could no longer fit into my favorite stylish black trousers. At that time I had taken a freelance position as a graphic designer in apparel. In almost two decades of working in that realm, I knew that the way you look and dress is everything and unconsciously you are judged for it. Because of this, I had always looked after myself and kept myself fit. Hence why, when the tire around my hips began expanding, it seemed very foreign to me.

THE JOURNEY BACK TO HEALTH

It was January 2021 and I was at my lowest point. I was feeling desperate and I made the decision to change. I was looking for a program that I could do to help me regain control over my weight and my health. I found a training program called 10X by Lorenzo Delano. It is a fascinating program wherein you work out 15 minutes twice per week and are able to maintain high levels of strength and fitness.

The first week in the program I purchased my pull-up bar. I secured it, or so I thought I did and I tested the bar a few times. I tied the black resistance band to the bar to aid my pull ups. With anticipation, I went to try it with my mother looking on. My mother watched as I placed my hands on the bar and my right foot on the resistance band. I tried to pull my upper body up. On my descent, time seemed to slow down as the bar fell. I felt like I was looking through my mother's horrified eyes as I crashed to the ground and fell into the abyss of the pain.

This was my second major physical trauma but just like the first time, I tried to minimize what had happened. I wasn't about to let this so-called hiccup get in the way of attaining my dream body. I took a few days off the workouts and during that week I took extensive actions to speed up the recovery. I was taking anti-inflammatory painkillers, turmeric supplements, applying ice packs, having an epsom salt bath every night and applying tiger balm before bed. To the naked eye it would seem to be just a lower back injury, however the months to come showed it was much more than that.

The pain seemed to get worse with each passing day. The evenings were the worst though, like a horror show. Somehow the pain would multiply itself and my nights turned into endless silent cries of pain. The pain would abruptly awaken me in the middle of the night, giving me little peace or rest, crying out over and over again.

My doctor had recommended taking medication to aid with the pain and suggested that I gradually increase the dose. He told me that this medication behaved as an antidepressant once the dose exceeded 60 mg. I decided to research the medication and found that the one of the possible side effects of the medication was that it "may induce suicide more than other antidepressants." I was desperate though, so I cautiously took a low dose of the medication. It numbed the extreme pain and made it tolerable.

I continued to take a low dose of the medicine every day and I resumed my 10X workouts. I watched my body transform to its best version and I rapidly lost the excess weight. My friends began noticing "Wow you've lost so much weight, you look amazing" and I felt really great. The 10X workouts had become my "Ultimate Medicine".

I got stronger day by day and I was getting back to myself. The 10X workouts had become a catalyst of hope and faith, a glimpse to a 100% recovery. Surely if my body could create such rapid transformation in my muscle mass and strength, surely it would create a faster recovery?

All I know right now is that I feel strong in my body, I have a body that I feel so proud of, regained my personal power and every time my biomechanist sees me he's impressed with the recovery and keeps telling me "keep doing that training you're doing — 10X".

I am not 100% recovered, but I would say above 85%. All I know right now is that the pudendal nerve (interestingly enough pudendal comes from a Latin word meaning, "to be ashamed" — a "behind the times" reference to the external genitalia) which runs between these two muscles; the piriformis and coccygeus are getting the maximum and rapid recovery through the 10X method.

I can finally walk my puppy for a long walk to the park without panic or extreme pain.

Life has definitely shown me how I took the essentials for granted — health and the basic full range of motion; sitting and walking.

If it hadn't been for the 10X method, who knows if I'd be writing this chapter today — it's given me the strength, hope and faith that I need today to face this ever evolving pelvic journey. To some it may just be a fitness workout, however when experiencing the whole physical body and health transformation, one has the potential to see themselves as an unstoppable human being with superhuman strength — with an inner strength and power to conquer any challenges in life.

If you are suffering from pain, I highly recommend the 10X Fitness Method. One, for rapid muscle recovery and two, to regain your personal power — the suffering has a way of making us feel powerless. Take back control today and don't shy away from pain, push through your mental barriers and achieve the unimaginable.

THE 10X METHOD

The 6X Alpha Routine is a great routine. This explosive and extraordinary workout will keep you at bay from loss of muscle mass and strength and will help you to preserve and increase your HealthSpan. For the optimal effect it is recommended to do the 6X Alpha routine as a 15 min workout twice a week.

The 6X Alpha routine consists of six exercises — six 10X sets — a full body workout stimulating the lower and upper body.

The 6X Alpha Routine:
Leg Press
The Pulldown
The Chest Press
Leg Press again or the Stiff-leg deadlift
The Row
The Overhead Press

Have fun with it!

FINAL NOTE

On a final note, as I am adding onto this chapter — on the 31st of August 2022, I've had a recent transformative breakthrough, a day I have begged, hoped and prayed for. The supplication of ending my suffering has finally been realized in my reality. With Resilience, Consistent Actions and Relentless Fight for my Sanity and Health — the day has arrived where I am 100% fully recovered. As I am writing this, my brain is still catching up to the physical breakthrough and I still can't quite believe it — when my Bio Mechanist said last week; "It's Gone". It's finally gone.

Keep calm and carry on.
~ WINSTON CHURCHILL

👤 ABOUT THE AUTHOR

Stéphanie is the Founder of Akashabe and created the Personal Power Life Method, after her frustrations of feeling powerless. The method uniquely combines Reiki, Kung Fu, Yoga, Shamanism and various other modalities and belief systems.

Stéphanie first became a Reiki Student and Practitioner. She then studied for her Yoga Teacher's Training in an Ashram after experiencing a burnout, leading her to seek answers through her self-discovery path. Stéphanie furthered her knowledge in India through a 500-hour Yoga Teacher's Training and then studied Shamanism, Life Coaching, Breath Coaching, the 10X Fitness Method and Holistic Health.

She is now a Certified 10X Fitness Coach, Health & Wellness Coach, Life Coach, Breath Coach, Yoga Teacher, Stretching Coach, a Reiki Practitioner, Author, Writer and Designer.

Stéphanie's Mission is to empower people with simple, effective tools to unleash their full potential in their day-to-day life and align with their empowered conscious self—their true self. Keep an eye out for her book, coming out in 2023.

Contact Information:

Websites:
https://stephaniescorial.com
https://akashabe.com

Social Media:
https://www.instagram.com/stephaniescorial/
https://www.instagram.com/akashabe/
https://www.linkedin.com/in/stephaniescorial/

A loving mother can quickly find her life is out of balance. It takes courage and strength to recognize her needs are as important as everyone else.

~Nadia Blackstock

The thing that is really hard, and really amazing, is giving up on being perfect and beginning the work of becoming yourself.

~Anna Quindlen

CHAPTER 13
SELF, FAMILY, WORK

by Nadia Blackstock

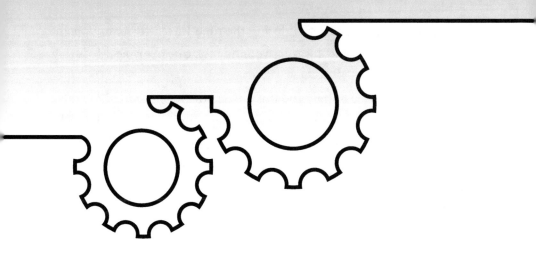

TOPIC: | Goal Setting & Creating a Plan For Optimal Physical Health

TOOL: | Gaining Clarity

TECHNIQUE: | Focus on new goals, nutrition and exercise

Clarity precedes success.

~ROBIN SHARMA

I successfully went from 203 pounds (92kg) down to 143 pounds (65kg) in six months and I have kept the weight off for over a year. I am sharing my story here because before this amazing health transformation, I would not have believed that it was possible for me to make such a massive change in such a short period of my time. I did it and I am motivated to share my story to inspire others and show them that they, too, can become the healthiest version of themselves.

I grew up in Australia and during the time I lived there, my weight remained relatively stable. I was active and I took care of my health during my early life.

In 2005, I moved to Italy and this is when the weight started to slowly creep on. When I moved to Italy, it was a huge change in my eating habits, as well as in the type of work I was doing and these lifestyle changes resulted in a long, steady weight increase. I eventually got married and had two children and my weight continued to increase. I gained a lot of weight with each pregnancy and it seemed like it was impossible to lose this pregnancy weight with all of my new responsibilities of caring for my two children on top of managing my career, my home and my life.

I was in a state of denial back then, I wasn't willing to take responsibility for my weight or my health. I used many excuses. "I can't help it, it's my genetics," "I don't have time, I'm a busy mom," "Exercise takes too much time," "Whenever I try to lose weight, I always fail," and "I just have to look at food and gain weight."

If there was an excuse, I made it. I could probably write an entire book of all the excuses I told myself! Maybe this resonates with you, maybe you recognize yourself in my story. It is the story of many of us. The story we are taught by society is that as we get older, it is natural to gain weight and lose some of the vibrancy of youth. We are taught that, we believe it and then we live by those beliefs. But justifying ourselves or making up excuses only leads to nothingness. No action! No change! No progress!

It wasn't just my excuses holding me back, though. It was my belief that being a good mother meant putting everyone else's needs before my own. We only have so many hours in a day, how could I make time for myself? And if I'm honest, the last thing I felt like doing was exercising or having to make one meal for myself and a separate meal for the rest of my family! I was overwhelmed and stressed and I dealt with that stress by eating. Chocolate was my favorite. Not the best coping mechanism, I know, but that's what I did. And with the chocolate, came the weight until that day when I reached my maximum weight of 203 pounds (92kg).

When you are overweight, or even obese like in my case, you always feel tired. You wake up every morning feeling like you need to go back to sleep. Everyday tasks are more difficult. You have very little energy or motivation. I wanted to be able to play with my children, to be able to go shopping and find clothes that actually looked nice and fit me, but I never made the time for those things. I had no balance in my life between myself, my family and my career. I didn't know how to change this but I was determined to do so.

I knew my weight was an issue. I had tried many diets in the past with little to no success, I felt defeated even before I started. I decided to get to the bottom of this and figure out why I was not able to stick to a diet. I started giving a lot of thought to why I had failed so much in the past. I realized it was my mindset that was the problem. I wasn't used to prioritizing myself. I didn't know how to take care of myself. I had spent so many years taking care of everybody but me that I no longer even knew what I wanted.

So I began to ask myself a series of questions.

I asked myself:

1. How do I want to look and feel?
2. What do I need to change?
3. Do I like my job?
4. Does my job provide the lifestyle I actually want?
5. Does my job give me fulfillment and satisfaction?

6. Does my lifestyle allow me to be there for my family and friends?
7. How do I want to show up?
8. What does being a good mum and wife really mean to me?

These questions gave me a clear target on what I needed to change and improve. I got very clear on who I was and what I wanted. I finally understood that working on myself first would actually help me be a better mom and a better wife. Working on myself ticked both boxes of self and family.

I made a commitment to work on myself. I took classes and learned about health and nutrition. I learned about mindfulness techniques to reduce my stress and tension. I began to see massive results and this spurred me to take even more action. Success breeds success.

Eventually, I decided that I wanted to share these new learnings with the people around me, so I began to counsel my friends and family on healthy lifestyle tips. This led me to realize that I would love to share my journey and the lessons I've learned with a bigger group of people, so I decided to get some health coaching certifications. Going on this journey to become a health coach has completely transformed my life. I wake up happy and energized each day, eager to share my knowledge and help people to create their best life. It has been an amazing journey and I am so glad that I finally got sick and tired of being sick and tired.

This is my health story and it can be yours too.

Below, I share my best tips for creating your own health transformation.

HOW TO CREATE A HEALTH TRANSFORMATION

Step 1: Gain Clarity and Take Responsibility

It's important to understand and recognize how you got to this point in your life. You must take full responsibility for your current state of health. Taking full responsibility will help you to make the commitment to create the necessary changes in your life. Once you have assumed responsibility, it is time to dream about what your ideal state of health would be and what you really want in your life. Gaining clarity around your goals will help you to construct a plan to move forward. Allow yourself to dream big and let yourself have the very highest aspirations for yourself.

Begin by going deep and asking yourself what you really want. You can use the questions below as a starting point to gain clarity around where you are today and how you got here as well as for creating a vision for the future.

Self Reflection Questions:

1. What is the current state of my health?
2. How is my weight, my cardiovascular fitness and my muscle tone?
3. How did I get here? What were the behaviors that caused me to be in the situation I am currently in?
   a. Examine diet, exercise, lifestyle choices, family dynamics and work atmosphere.
   b. What type of people do you spend the most time with and are they healthy and happy?
4. What level of activity do I currently do?
5. What does my ideal vision for the future look like?
6. If I had the body that I dream of, what would that look like?
   a. What weight would you be?
   b. How would your body look?
   c. What kind of clothing would you wear?
   d. What would be your level of cardiovascular fitness and muscle tone?
7. Ideally, what form of exercise would be sustainable and enjoyable?
8. What is my ideal job?
9. What would my ideal family relationships look like? Do I currently have that?

10. What type of friends would I like to have to support my active lifestyle? What type of friends would encourage me and inspire me and support me best?

11. What is my mission here? If I could leave the world with one lesson, one thing I stood for, what would it be?

Answer these questions and any other questions that will help you to gain clarity around your past and your hopes for the future. Be very honest with yourself here and allow yourself the luxury of dreaming your biggest dreams for yourself. What would the ideal version of you look like?

Step 2: Change Your Goal!

It is essential to pay close attention to your goals as far as health is concerned. When I first went on my journey, I realized I had the wrong goal. I always wanted to be thinner or to look better, but I realized that I could support myself better if I simply changed my goal. Instead of looking at a number on the scale and wishing for a different number, I decided to create a more powerful goal. I decided to have vibrant health be my goal.

So take a moment now and change your goal. What would be a great goal you can use that will really inspire change in your life? Instead of putting pressure on yourself to weigh yourself and aim for a lower number, figure out what goal would seriously motivate you. You need to have a powerful goal. One that is worth fighting for, full of desire, emotion and power over you. The outcome has to be a strong enough motivation to move you when your motivation starts to wither.

For me, that goal was vibrant health. Beyond that, I wanted vibrant health so that I could play with my two very active boys without feeling like I am about to drop! I want to avoid getting the illnesses like diabetes, alzheimers and cancer that my grandparents had died from. I want to have the possibility of living a long, healthy life with my family. These are all things I will always want and will never give up on.

So what is your goal? What would make you feel excited to get healthy? Do you want a sexy body to feel good in clothing? Or maybe you want to be attractive and sexy for your lover. Is it that you want to stay active and participate in fun hobbies? Maybe you want to be healthy so that you can feel good. Perhaps you, like me, want to avoid the generational illnesses that have plagued your family. Or you might just want to be a good role model for your children, spouse, family, friends or coworkers. Whatever your reason is, write it down on a piece of paper and post it on the bathroom mirror so you can read it at least twice a day when you brush your teeth.

When being healthy is your goal, it remains your goal for life! It changes your perspective on all your choices and actions. This is why I was able to lose all of that weight and reach my healthy weight for my age and height and I haven't struggled to keep it off. When being healthy is your goal, you start thinking about what your body wants, you show yourself love, you connect more within. One of the most powerful things you can do is start talking with your body, view it as one of your children, show it the same love and care you show them.

Step 3: Nutrition

It is time to create a diet that will support your body completely. Instead of dropping into the diet culture, aim to create a healthy meal plan that you can maintain.

Most diets are not sustainable. They are full of foods people rarely ever eat or don't like. Many diets are extremely restrictive and difficult to follow. To follow these types of diets often means having to search for all sorts of ingredients, take a lot of extra time to prepare, or require you to cook one meal for yourself and a totally different meal for your family. It is very difficult to maintain these diets. They feel like a punishment and sooner or later we give up.

The other issue with dieting is that even if you do actually manage to stick it out and you are able to follow the diet for as long as needed to reach your goal, you typically stop eating this way after you reach it. Then what do you do? You go back to your old habits. Those are the same habits that led you to gain weight in the first place. So without a doubt, the weight comes back. That's why knowing how you got to this point in the first place is so important.

Mindfully look at what you and your family eat, write everything down. If you are a parent like me, you probably cook the same meals each week. Children don't like change, they like to have the same food they are used to. This is good news because since you already know the meals that work for your family, you can tweak them slightly to make them healthier.

Take note of how hungry you are before and after each meal. Eat slowly and stop eating when you are full. Don't overeat. Refrain from feeling like you must finish everything on your plate. This is often a learned habit, left over from our childhoods, especially if we were raised with the mentality that we shouldn't waste food. By eating slowly and paying attention to how you feel, you can stop eating when you are full.

When snacking, ask yourself questions like:

- Am I really hungry?"
- Am I just eating for the sake of eating?
- Is it out of an emotional reason (boredom, sadness, stress)?
- Is it because I saw someone else eating (even on tv)?

Paying attention to why you are snacking can be a very easy way to decrease the amount of unnecessary food you are consuming. Typically, we snack on foods that are less nutritious so if you notice you are snacking because you truly are hungry, make sure you have healthy snacks on hand.

When you begin to focus on your food, aim to eat whole, nutritious foods. Avoid processed foods as much as possible. If you have a diet with a lot of processed foods, begin by simply looking at the ingredient list of the foods you are choosing. Notice if it is full of added sugar or refined flour.

In the beginning, simply aim to educate yourself. Learn what ingredients the processed food you are eating contain. Don't change anything at first. Once you understand what ingredients your food contains, aim to eliminate the least healthy foods first. Do this slowly, over time and be patient with yourself. Processed foods have a lot of salt, sugar and added fats, so they are not always easy to remove from our diets since our bodies have come to depend on them. Slowly reduce until most of the foods you are eating are natural, as close to the form they would be in nature as possible.

Eating healthy also means taking note of what is good for you. It is helpful to keep a food diary in the beginning to take note of how you feel directly after eating and the next day. Take note of anything you feel in your body. Are you noticing any swelling in your fingers or toes? Does your stomach feel bloated? What is your digestion like? See if you can notice how certain foods make you feel. Pay particular attention when eating foods like dairy, wheat and processed foods.

Remember that every person is different. What is healthy for me is not necessarily healthy for other people. Even foods that many of us consider healthy can be detrimental to your body. Each of us must determine what diet works best for us. Act like a detective to discover what works for you.

If you suspect that a particular food is not working for you, eliminate it from your diet for two weeks. Then reintroduce the food and pay close attention to how you feel after you eat as well as the following day. This is the easiest way to find out if your body is reacting badly to certain foods. Nutritious foods that work for you will keep you feeling full for longer and you will not have digestive problems, or any inflammation like bloating or swelling. When your diet is working for you, you feel great, filled with energy and ready to face anything. A good diet even affects your mood, so pay attention to all the physical signs as you craft your perfect personalized diet.

Once you start feeling the benefits of eating healthy, you don't want to stop. Food becomes a natural feel-good drug. When you do eat something not good for you, your body soon lets you know about it. Eating healthy will support your new, more healthy body and give you the energy to create the life you dream of.

Step 4: Exercise!

Now that you have gained clarity, found a new, more powerful goal and created a new nutrition plan, it is time to turn to exercise.

If you don't love to exercise, don't worry, I was once where you are. I used to hate to exercise, but now I understand that it is a key element for creating a healthy body and a healthy life. Even better, once you start moving, you will feel great!

There is no getting around it. Our bodies were made to move, we need to move on a regular basis. The good thing is that a little goes a long way, but you must be consistent. To make sure, you can't leave it to chance. Set a time of day for it and schedule it into your to do list, giving it the same importance you give to other things you have scheduled.

There are many different exercise programs available in the gym or online. The possibilities are endless really. If I have to exercise, I want to do it in a way that is fun! If you choose something you enjoy, or at least do it with people you have fun with, it becomes easier to do. Some forms of exercise give you better results than others, such as strength and resistance training, but it is essential in the beginning to pick an activity that is something that you enjoy and will keep on doing. You can pick one activity or a few different activities to mix it up a bit.

Step 5: Self Love & Compassion

Another extremely important step toward success and finding balance is viewing your body and treating yourself with the same love and compassion that you treat your children and other people you love. Refrain from being overly critical of yourself when you slip up and make a mistake. There will always be that day when you are too physically tired to do your scheduled exercise for the day, or the day when you give into a food craving. It's only natural, so accept those moments with love and grace. Give yourself permission to be imperfect. Remember, you are perfectly imperfect! We all are.

FINAL WORDS

In the end, changing your approach to health will help you to create a system that works for you. Once you change your goal to one of focusing on health, you can tailor your nutrition, your exercise and your mindset to support your goals.

As for me, when I changed my goal to being focused on health, I improved the way I felt, I increased my self esteem and improved my confidence. This has made me a better mother, a better wife and a better person. I have changed so many things and I have felt so uplifted by the path I have taken that I have become a holistic health coach. I now have a career that fills my life with joy and satisfaction while still having the time and energy to be fully present for my family.

Now as a certified health coach, I want to help all those out there who relate to my story and need support to find their personal balance between self, family and work. You don't have to do it on your own either. Having the help of family members, friends or a coach can really make a huge difference.

So don't hold off. Start your transformation now.

TIPS TO REMEMBER

- Become mindful
- Stop making excuses
- Choose a goal that is realistic, achievable and full of emotion, like the goal of health
- Show yourself the same love and compassion that you have for your children and other loved ones
- Make food preparation as easy as possible
- Eat slowly and stop when you feel full
- Listen to your body
- Become consistent with exercise and make it fun
- Never forget you are important
- Show yourself the same kind of love that you give to those you love

Wellness is a connection of paths: knowledge and action.

~JOSHUA HOLTZ

ABOUT THE AUTHOR

Nadia Blackstock is a Certified Holistic Health and Fitness Coach. She was born and raised in Australia. In 2005, she decided to move to Italy and work as an ESL teacher where she soon met her husband, had two children and gained over 30kg. After dramatically improving her health and fitness, she decided to make a career change and studied to become a certified Holobody, 10X Fitness and Level 1 Precision Nutrition Health Coach.

She understands that transformation is a delicate process and unique to each and every one of us. That is why when you work with her, she creates a tailor made program, identifying where you currently are, what obstacles and challenges you are facing and what goals you want to obtain.

Nadia's personal goal now is to help 1000 other mothers over the next 5 years attain their natural balance between family, self and work.

Contact Information:
nadia@nadiablackstock.com
www.nadiablackstock.com
https://www.linkedin.com/in/nadia-blackstock
https://www.instagram.com/nadiablackstock.healthcoach/

**Let Food Be Thy Medicine,
Thy Medicine Shall Be Thy Food.**

~Hippocrates

CHAPTER 14
A SUPPORTIVE MEAL PLAN
by Karla Ornelas

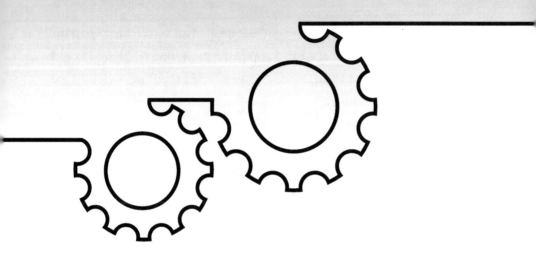

TOPIC:	Nutrition
TOOL:	A Healthy Meal Plan
TECHNIQUE:	Focus on hydration and nutrition to move towards peak health.

The Doctor Of The Future Will No Longer Treat The Human Frame With Drugs, But Rather Will Cure And Prevent Disease With Nutrition.

~THOMAS EDISON

As a child, I was skinny. I have memories of people who would encourage me to eat more because I was all skin and bones. Later on, as a teenager, I got into rowing and dancing and I actually built a rather striking figure. I had an hourglass shape and I was complimented for it all the time, I was no longer encouraged to "eat more", rather I began getting questions on how I did it. I could honestly answer that I trained six days a week, but the truth is that being thin was my nature.

At nineteen I left home for university. I had all sorts of new responsibilities once I got to school and I also had a newfound freedom. I could eat when and how I wanted. Since I never worried about my weight, I ate anything and everything.

At around this time, I got really sick with hepatitis. Until then, I did not enjoy sugar at all, I barely tolerated sweet things. I would take the frosting off the cake because it was unbearable. That all changed when I got hepatitis. For some reason, the doctors I saw when I got sick recommended that I eat candy in order to heal. I know, it seems counterintuitive, but that's what they said. So I started eating candy. Now, you may not be aware of this, but the only way to develop a taste for sweets is by eating sweets. The proverbial sugar monster in me was born during my hepatitis convalescence.

That was the moment everything changed for me. As I ate sugar to satisfy my ever growing need for sweets, I began to gain weight. I paid little to no attention to the ingredients in the food I was eating and began to take in sugar multiple times every day.

I continued to work out, but not as intensely as I had during high school. My sleep began to be affected and my sleeping patterns were often disrupted. It was at this point that stress began to be a factor.

One day when I was home from university, my mom told me that I had gained weight. I had to be told, because even if my clothes didn't fit quite the same, I really did not know what was happening. Being overweight was an entirely new experience for me. I hadn't even realized it was happening. This was when my yo-yo dieting ordeal began. And it would be a feature of my life for the next twenty-some years.

In 2019, I was putting on a pair of shorts that had fit quite well the last time I had seen them and I noticed that they were hard to put on. I know many of you have had this experience. You know the scenario. You can't put your pants on so you lie flat on your back on the bed and suck your tummy in, in order to get the zipper to go all the way up. That's what it took that day to get my shorts on. I was laughing at myself but for some reason, the experience stuck with me. I thought about it a lot over the next few days and I decided I needed to change something.

I found the nerve to make a promise to myself. I decided that I would never, ever have to do this sucking in my belly to fit into my clothes again. I would lose the extra weight and I would never let myself get like this again. I decided that those shorts would be my measure. I will never let myself be lying on the bed again to zip them up. It was a solemn promise I made to myself.

Have you ever been there? Maybe you've promised yourself something similar many times. We all have.

I myself had made promises like this before but this time it was different for me. I knew this because this time, the promise came from the deepest recesses of my heart. I made that promise with tears in my eyes and a knot in my throat. Maybe I should describe it as the whisper of my soul. I just felt it with all my being. I will never, ever, get like this again.

I did not know it at that time, but when the despair is so deep and your mind and heart are in consonance with what you want, the answers come to you. Many are the names for this, synchronicity, law of attraction, serendipity, right place-right time, the universe answering, the YouTube algorithm. Whatever it is, it works.

The thing is, that shortly after that day, I began getting ads from a personal growth platform and one that jumped out at me was a program called Wildfit. I learned about the program by watching a masterclass on YouTube and it made sense to me. I realized I had not been taking care of myself or eating right for the past two decades. I had been hating my body and "its tendency to gain weight" when the reality was that my body was just responding to the input that I, *myself* and *no one else*, had been giving it.

I decided to enroll in the full program and it was amazing. I was very serious as I followed the program and I got very valuable lessons that began my transformation. It didn't stop there though. Once I began to learn, I didn't want to stop. I began to learn everything I could about diet and nutrition and I incorporated this information into my life. I changed the food I eat, but also the frequency with which I eat. Changing my food habits has had the largest impact regarding not only my weight, but also my health. I call the way I eat today my Supportive Meal Plan.

This Supportive Meal Plan combines a number of the lessons that I have learned along the way and the magic of it is that I fit it into my lifestyle, my preferences, my tastes and my values. Yes, there are some things that changed a lot from the way I ate before, but the changes were not that difficult, because they were either gradual, small or just so clearly useful that going back to how it was before was no longer an option.

I will now describe the main building blocks of the Supportive Meal Plan. I have come to realize that everyone can combine these elements to create their own plans that fit in with their own lifestyle and that will bring them to a healthier physique.

Element 1: Hydration

The first element is to have proper hydration. Drinking enough water is indispensable for our organs and cells to work properly. How much water we should drink every day varies from one person to the next, but a good rule of thumb is around two liters. Depending on our level of activity, the weather and a few other factors, we may need some more. It is important to realize that water is essential to our health and water is the best way to hydrate.

Element 2: Nutrition

There is a lot of misguiding, confusing and overtly false information about nutrition and "healthy food" available. It is challenging to figure out for certain what is and what isn't healthy. My guiding light in sorting through all the misinformation is to stay closer to the diet that humans have evolved with.

Sugar

Sugar should only be a rare occurrence in our meals. The good news is that as much as eating more sweets makes one crave more sweets, eating less sweets makes us crave it less. The difficulty here is that sugar is in pretty much every processed food available in our markets. Therefore, reducing the amount of processed foods and increasing the amount of whole foods is a great way to eliminate a huge amount of the added sugar in our diet. If possible, aim to cook your food from scratch as much as possible. This will be the best way to be in control of the amount of sugar you take in.

Intermittent Fasting

The body takes energy and time to digest and process the nutrients in our food, time being the key word here. The more time one allows between meals for your body to do what it doesn't. For this, consider intermittent fasting as an option. With intermittent fasting, you set a time where you don't eat each day, called the feeding window and the rest of the time you fast. You can experiment with what works for you in terms of how many hours to fast each day. Since each of us is different, it is important to find what works for you.

If intermittent fasting seems extreme to you, consider that you most likely already do a form of intermittent fasting. If you are eating between 9 AM and 8 PM as most people do, you currently have a 13-11 schedule where you are fasting for 13 hours and eating for 11. If you want to try intermittent fasting, slowly, over time, increase your fasting window until you find one that works for you. It is essential to get all of the vitamins and nutrients you need during your feeding window, so make sure you are eating healthy and getting nutrient dense calories.

Protein

Protein is the most important nutrient for our health. Protein combines well with fat or with carbohydrates, but mixing carbohydrates and fats is not functional for our bodies. You can eat in a way that you mix proteins with fats for a few days and then switch to protein and carbohydrates for a few days. Alternatively, you can switch each day from one mixing technique to another.

I have found that my body works best when I eat the same nutrients for a few days in a row. This means that I eat protein with fats for two to three days in a row and then I eat protein with carbohydrates for another two to three days in a row. I eat in this pattern and it works great for me but I only learned this after experimenting with different methods of combining foods.

It is imperative to figure out for yourself what works for you. Just as one method works for me, other methods work for other people. I know plenty of people who find that switching every other day works for them perfectly.

Focus on nutrient dense foods like green vegetables in order to become healthier and stay lean. You could even add green smoothies to your daily routine in order to ensure that you are getting all of the vitamins and nutrients that you need. Green smoothies are a great way to add whole foods into your diet. If you have never had a green smoothie before, it may seem a bit weird, but once you find a recipe that works for you, you may find that a green smoothie is one of the greatest things you can do for your health.

PERSONALIZE YOUR FOOD PLAN

Once you start discovering which foods work for you and which foods don't, it is essential that you create a sustainable plan of action for your nutrition. It is wise to go very slowly in the beginning, implementing one small change at a time and letting it settle in before you move on to the next change. Small changes done consistently over time yield the best results. The key to success will be personalizing your meal plan to work for your body and your lifestyle. Once you find the right combination of foods, you will feel great, which helps to maintain the system. Keep learning about nutrition and put the knowledge to work for you. Take your time to create the best possible meal plan for you.

I personally designed my own meal plan by bringing together all the knowledge I gained during this journey. It has been easy for me to stick to it and keep myself slender because I feel amazing and I know it is because of my healthy diet. I do still fall off the wagon but when I do, I have compassion for myself and I jump back into my meal plan as soon as I can.

Another key aspect is forgiving yourself for the past habits you had and choices you made. Forgiving yourself may just be the most powerful gift you can give yourself. Set yourself free from the judgment you may have heaped upon yourself. For me, it has been very powerful to forgive myself for my messy eating habits and for the awful words I used to say to myself. It took me time and many tears, to understand that my weight problem was a part of my self-love problem.

FINAL WORDS

During my journey, I dropped the excess weight that I had struggled with for so long. I can zip up those shorts, while standing up and even puffing my tummy out a bit. And most importantly I know that my journey to becoming slender again, has also been a journey of self-love. Today, I am able to look at myself in the mirror and say truly and deeply "I love myself".

And if I could do it, so can you.

I hope that you go forward with the knowledge that weight issues can be overcome, by learning about food and nutrition and then putting it into practice. And, of course, by loving, loving, loving yourself.

Please reach out to me if you would like to share your healing journey. I would love to hear from you.

~Karla

The soul always knows what to do to heal itself.
The challenge is to silence the mind.
~ CAROLINE MYSS

ABOUT THE AUTHOR

Karla Ornelas began her self-love journey in 2016, as a means of getting out of a depression without using medication. She has not only overcome depression, but has also transformed her physique and begun a spiritual journey.

Although she has a day job, in her spare time she enjoys helping other people on their own journeys. To that end, she works with Akashic records and is a certified Mindvalley Holobody and 10x Coach.

Contact Info:

Email at karlatol@hotmail.com

PART 3
LIFESTYLE CHOICES: DAILY ROUTINES

If we could give every individual the right
amount of nourishment and exercise,
not too little and not too much, we
would have the safest way to health.

~ HIPPOCRATES

PART 3: LIFESTYLE CHOICES: DAILY ROUTINES

What is the best way to get started on your journey towards ultimate health and wellness? You start with your daily habits.

Daily habits, done consistently, will lead to huge lifestyle shifts. Installing new habits may take some time but they are well worth the effort. The greatest thing about habits is that once you create the habit, it becomes automatic. Once established, it takes very little to maintain. That is the beauty of habit.

The funny thing is that each one of us already has a lot of habits. Unfortunately, many of these habits are unhealthy. For instance, do you hit your snooze button repeatedly and wind up getting up so late that you have to race around to get everything you need done? Do you grab food from a fast food restaurant and end up making poor choices? Do you get home and immediately plunk yourself down on your couch and then spend the evening zoned out snacking and watching television? If so, you are doing habitual activities that you have become accustomed to.

The good news is that we can decide to do something different. We can choose to add new habits to our days and nights so that we can begin to create a better life and better health for ourselves. Day by day you add small, simple changes until eventually, you are living a totally different life.

It doesn't have to be difficult to create extraordinary health. The stories on the following pages will show you how to add simple daily habits to your life that will help you optimize your day so that you are embracing a healthy lifestyle instead of trying to force it. Imagine rising early each day and starting your day with a nourishing morning routine. Or learning to embrace discipline as a daily practice. Or installing daily routines where healthy eating and exercise are woven throughout your day. This is the way to create a life of health and wellness.

Let's do it. Let's add some healthy habits into your life.

The first step to win yourself is to wake up early.

~Sukant Ratnakar

CHAPTER 15

EARLY RISING FOR HEALTH AND BALANCE

by Aviram Trachtenberg

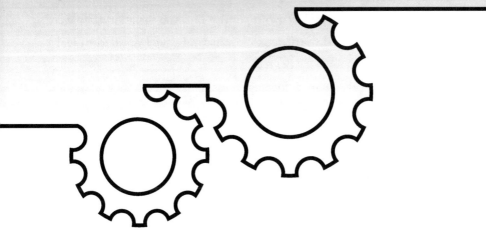

TOPIC:	Healthy Habits
TOOL:	Early Rising
TECHNIQUE:	Commit to waking up early in order to start your day right. If you really want to commit to the early wake up, join the 5 AM club and watch your life transform.

Work hard, stay positive and get up early.
It's the best part of the day.

~ GEORGE ALLEN

For my entire life I was interested in health and nutrition. I was always very active when I was younger and I enjoyed sports such as swimming, martial arts and basketball. Although I was always very active, I was also overweight as a teen and it bothered me that these activities did not help maintain a normal weight.

Looking at my surroundings and seeing many members of my family overweight got me into nutrition and health. I guess subconsciously I wanted to help them, as well as avoid getting into the situation they were in as I got older. I found nutrition so fascinating that I decided to learn food science for my bachelor's degree.

I had been working in a meat processing factory and understood that this was not the job of my dreams, which is why I was committed to getting an education so I could get a better job as an adult. During my college years, I studied hard and began exploring and researching health and disease. I had a particular interest in cancer and leukemia. I feel that I was drawn into those studies because I have a grandmother that I never got to meet. She died from leukemia before I was born. My dissertation was on acute myeloid leukemia and the potential of plant-derived phenolic compounds to abolish the leukemic cells. I eventually completed my college years and graduated with a Ph.D. in health science.

As you can see, knowledge was not the problem. I had all of this formal education and yet, I still found it difficult to apply it in real life. I wondered why I couldn't be an energetic person with a beautiful body; I thought it must be my heredity, my lot in life and I just accepted that I would never be able to transform my body.

During these years, I had a lot of beliefs that were not very helpful to me. I believed that since everyone in my family was overweight, it must run in my family. I thought that since I was young, I could eat whatever I wanted because my body could handle it.

I also held beliefs about people who were healthy and in great shape. I believed that all these people with beautiful bodies were clearly sacrificing their life for it. I figured they were not eating what they wanted to eat, or that they were depriving themselves by eating very little food, or perhaps they were going to the gym 5 times a week. I remember thinking that I would never want to live that way, that this way of living was not for me. These beliefs kept me exactly where I was.

When the worldwide pandemic began, I was overweight, lazy and on a path towards a lifetime of ill health. I would come home from work, take care of the kids, eat dinner and then finish my evening by watching TV in bed with snacks. I was on a bad path. Something had to change.

One day, I found a personal transformation program and decided to check it out. The program was really transformative for me because I hadn't worked on myself for years. This experience was so great that it set me on a path of learning that I am still on to this day. I have read so many books, done a ton of online courses and listened to endless podcasts on various areas of personal growth. I felt my mindset shifting.

The process changed my perspective in every part of my life, including my health. The first thing that changed were my beliefs. When I examined the beliefs I held I quickly realized they were detrimental to me. They were in direct opposition to creating a healthy lifestyle. It became clear that my beliefs hampered my ability to install a healthier way of living. This was the moment that I knew I had to change.

And so it began. I started by replacing my negative beliefs with more empowering ones. I wrote an amazing vision for the way I wanted to be in the future. I created the grandest version of my future self and I held onto that vision. I also thought about why I wanted to attain this vision and this helped me to create a powerful reason for transforming my life. My reason was simple: I wanted to be healthy so I could become the very best version of myself and that would enable me to live the very best life possible. Then it was time to create the plan. Armed with all my new personal growth tools, I developed a strategy for making my vision a reality. I was ready.

Once I acquired the inner knowledge of where I wanted to be, I became very motivated. I was able to change many parts of my life so that I could reach my goals. My mindset shift had been profound, because I now knew what I needed to do to create the life I dreamed of. Every single day I worked with consistency and it slowly brought the change I had desired. The transformation was not immediate but as time went on, I noticed how much more energy I had and how much better I felt. Although the change took time, it happened faster than I believed possible. After a lifetime of being overweight and fighting my body, I was finally making progress. It was amazing.

THE 5 AM CLUB

The secret; for me, the one thing that changed my health the most, was when I learned about the 5 AM Club. This is a concept pioneered by Robin Sharma, where he advocates for awakening at 5 AM every day. The theory is that when you wake up that early, you are able to get things accomplished before your day even starts. The super early wake-up time creates a space where you can take care of yourself first. This motivates you and energizes you so that you can more easily create the life you want.

I decided that I would try it. I began by waking up at 5 AM every morning. This habit brought a lot of power and energy to me. I was able to take care of myself first and this allowed me to take care of everything else I needed to after that.

The theory is the same as the reason that when you are on an airplane, the instructions are that in case of emergency you are to put the oxygen mask on yourself first. The idea is that you cannot help anyone else if you yourself are not in a good place.

Just as I would put my oxygen mask on in an emergency on an airplane, I wake up at 5 AM so that I can take care of myself first. When I first started to do this, I didn't want to do what I usually did every morning. I didn't want to just begin my day earlier and start drinking coffee and scrolling through my social media. That never made me feel good and I knew that it was not a great way to take care of myself. Instead, I chose to utilize my mornings to give myself a strong jumpstart to my day.

MORNING ROUTINE

I decided that I would take an hour each morning to take care of myself. I split my mornings into 3 sections of 20 minutes each. I meditate, exercise and spend time reading or journaling.

My mornings begin with a big glass of water with a pinch of Himalayan salt to rehydrate my body. During the night we lose a lot of water, so rehydration is essential. Next, I meditate so I can start my day with a sense of calm, which prolongs the Alpha brain wave frequency - a more relaxed state of mind. After meditation, I exercise. This might be yoga, running or walking outside, or resistance training. Moving early in the morning produces good hormones and biochemicals, bringing a great boost of energy. I also make sure that I either read a chapter in a book, listen to a podcast, or journal so that I can exercise my mind.

During my morning routine, I am essentially taking care of my body, mind and spirit! It is a great way to start the day. After this amazing session, I am ready to go about my day, facing any challenge with a smile. I appreciate my mornings even more when I am lucky enough to catch a beautiful sunrise through the window, or spend a few minutes outside every day before I go to work. Prior to this new habit of awakening so early, I rarely saw the sunrise.

Establishing this habit for me was pretty simple, as at the time my newborn daughter woke me up before 5 AM, so I just stayed awake and it stuck. But most of us don't have these circumstances, so to start practicing waking up earlier, begin with small steps. For the first few days, simply wake up a few minutes earlier than usual and use that time to do something that makes you happy. Whether that means you meditate or listen to music or sit outside for a few minutes, make sure it is something you really enjoy. As time goes on, continue to wake up earlier and earlier until you are waking up early enough to have a really nice morning routine. You can call this your power hour to make it feel even more special.

Why should you wake up early? Well, biologically we are meant to rise when the sun comes up and go to bed when the sun goes down. Melatonin is the sleep hormone which controls the sleep-wake cycle. Melatonin rises when it is dark and drops when the cells in our retina receive sunlight. We are naturally attuned to being more responsive and alert in the morning and drowsy and sleepy at night.

Some exciting new research shows that people that prefer to do mental and physical activity later in the day are consistently found with poorer scores in all aspects of well-being when compared to people that prefer activities earlier in the day. Results from sleep-wake research shows that people who work best in the morning are healthier, less prone to cardiovascular disease, psychiatric symptoms, over consumption of carbs, obesity, diabetes and even cancer compared to their evening type counterparts.

Additionally, morning people were found to be more proactive as their biological alignment fits neatly with social time demands such as school and work schedules, Moreover, morning people were also found to be happier as a whole. These are some of the reasons you should consider waking up earlier, especially if you are an evening type individual.

IDENTITY SHIFT

How do you maintain waking up early to engage in self care? How do you make sure these habits become a part of your everyday routine? Well, it all comes down to changing your identity. By making your new identity one that prioritizes health and wellness, you will be able to easily add habits like waking up early so that you can take care of yourself. Identity shift is so important because exercising, eating well and installing new habits is no longer something you do but a part of who you are. Identity shift is a true game changer.

The shift should be gradual as you incorporate the new habits you want to bring in, like waking early. Before you know it, you will be doing many things to enhance your health. This may include exercising, doing yoga or stretching, practicing gratitude, dancing, listening to uplifting content, learning something new, reading a book, spending time outdoors or watching the sunrise or the sunset each day. Create an identity where these activities are simply part of who you are.

FINAL WORDS

After implementing the 5 AM club routine and other habits, I have had a huge transformation. Today I am proud to say that I have released 44 pounds (20 kgs), went from a body mass index of 28.4 to 21 and best of all, am very fit with 80% muscle tissue. I finally have the body that I dreamt of and I am able to maintain it easily.

My identity shifted slowly and I am now at the point where every day I am meditating, exercising, practicing gratitude, reading and learning something new. I really feel I am living an extraordinary life. I have two beautiful children and together with my beautiful wife that I love dearly, we created a home where we co-elevate each other and let each other fly in the direction of our dreams.

We travel as a family, camping in nature, staying at hotels, having adventures. We laugh a lot, but we are also goal-oriented, looking to achieve our life vision. My life has completely transformed in every way and I am thankful for everything that I accomplished. For me, the key to my transformation was waking up early. By joining the 5 AM club, I was able to create this amazing life I am now living. If I had not started waking up this early, I would not have had the time or energy to make the changes I needed to make to move from an ordinary, health degrading state to an extraordinary life of health and happiness.

I know that if you decide to implement the 5 AM club routine you will find many benefits that will manifest quicker than you think. However, even if you simply choose to wake up a little bit earlier than before so that you can do one thing that nourishes you, you will have a positive change in your life.

My personal journey has inspired me to do even more. I am now ready to help other people to transform into the best version of themselves. I am a certified health and fitness coach and I have already helped several people. I am teaching people how they too can lose weight by changing their relationship with their body and changing their perspective on how they should treat themselves. I have enjoyed this so much and I have realized that helping others on their health journey is something that I would do even if I didn't do it for a living. This is my mission and it is the best thing I can do for other people. I enjoy every moment of it. I am now living my best life and for me, it was all because I decided to begin waking up early and start my day with self care.

I have done it and so can you. If you are interested in learning more or in sharing your health journey with me, please reach out to me.

~Aviram

You've got to get up every morning with determination if you're going to go to bed with satisfaction.

~ GEORGE LORIMER

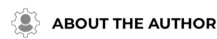

ABOUT THE AUTHOR

Aviram Trachtenberg from Israel, Ph.D. in health science and founder of Healthshely where he serves as a health and fitness coach. He is excited about transforming people's health by applying his knowledge and experience. He wants everyone to experience healthy living. The basis of his coaching centers around helping people to change their mindset and install new healthy habits. He loves teaching people his method, called "The Experience of Health and Wellness."

Contact Information:
healthshelyat@gmail.com
Website: www.healthshely.com
Instagram: aviramtberg
Facebook: Life itself club

There is something magical about the early morning.
It's a time when the world belongs to
only those few who are awake.
And we walk around like kings while
others remain unseen in their beds.

~Shawn Blanc

CHAPTER 16

A ROLLERCOASTER RIDE

by Aaron Eisner

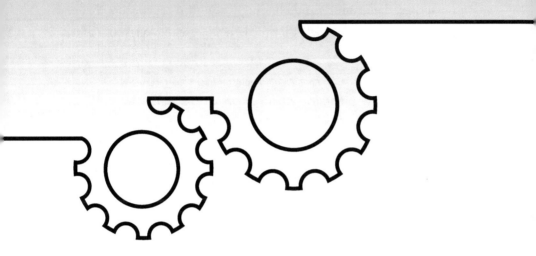

TOPIC:	Peak Performance & Habits
TOOL:	Morning Routine
TECHNIQUE:	Create a healthy early morning routine.

You'll never change your life until you
change something you do daily.
The secret of your success is found in your daily routine.

~JOHN C. MAXWELL

Sooner or later we all need to surrender to the fact that life is a long, crazy rollercoaster ride that elevates you from unimaginable heights, turns left and right and often even upside down and more often than we like, takes us by surprise. But in the end, if someone would ask me: "Would you like to take the easy ride, good scenery all the way through and a soft, but little dull ending, or would you like to take the crazy ride with all the ups and downs, turns and surprises, dark tunnels and blindingly beautiful experiences that ends on a powerful note?" One ticket for the latter, please. No questions asked.

> *Life should not be a journey to the grave*
> *with the intention of arriving safely*
> *in a pretty and well preserved body, but rather*
> *to skid in broadside in a cloud of smoke,*
> *thoroughly used up, totally worn out, and loudly proclaiming*
> *"Wow! What a Ride!*

~ HUNTER S. THOMPSON

While there is a healthy amount of luck in life, each of us has a good amount of power over which ride we choose, how and where we steer and with whom we want to ride. It was something of a revelation when I first realized that I have the power to design my own unique ride. For me, that moment began not too long after I finished my A-levels in Germany when I was just 18 years old.

I was reading a book called the *Code of the Extraordinary Mind* by Vishen Lakhiani. I remember nodding constantly while reading and feeling stunned as the truth of the words sank into me, as if the call to take responsibility for my own rollercoaster ride was in me all along. It was at that time when I woke up and decided that I can and will create a life that is extraordinary. That my intuitive feeling of bombarding everything and everyone around me with truth-seeking questions is actually the right way to go. And that there is a hell of a ride just waiting for me to say: "Count me in, baby!"

Now, four years later, my life has progressed into an exhilarating ride, changing me many times over. I am living a life where I travel and attend amazing events where I meet incredible people and I am on the path towards an amazing life. I look back gratefully on the fact that I had the courage to decide early in my life that I will take the crazy rollercoaster ride. In fact, I feel taken aback to ask myself: "Aaron, how did you brave your path up until now, scratches and scars displayed, to be the courageous man you are right now?"

I don't mean that I am perfect. In fact, I am far from it. Just at the time of writing, I am hanging upside down in my rollercoaster, doing my best to navigate my overwhelm as I juggle more challenges than ever in my life, trying to build my business while ending a soul crushing history of porn addiction. But I would say that I have, little by little, built myself into a person that believes in himself and has accumulated an effective toolbox that can take him sky high at the best while allowing him to keep his head above the water at the worst.

The most essential tool in this toolbox is my morning routine. And this is what I will delight you with in this brief time that you are reading this chapter, hoping that I can inspire you to build a morning practice that will leave you able to always stay above the water and also enable you to have your head in the clouds from time to time. Like a daily anchor to keep you on track.

And while everyone's ride looks different, we can still use the same tools and focus on one of the most essential things in life: our body. Because in the end, we need to realize that our body is the wagon that drives our rollercoaster. Better to have a body that fuels your dreams rather than dulls them. Are you ready?

MORNING ROUTINE

Wait, but I am not a morning person!

Good point.

It is indeed the case that some people are natural "night owls". However, if you have the capability to comfortably push your bedtime a little earlier or start your workday a little later, I would recommend embracing instituting a morning routine. There really is truth in the saying "win the morning and you win the day". So even if your time window in the morning is small, I am certain that you can build a powerful morning routine for yourself. This is a matter of prioritization of what matters to you in life. You are the artisan. Choose wisely.

Another important thing that we should get sorted before building your routine is the realization that you need to help yourself first before you can help others. This is a key insight to building, growing and maintaining a powerful morning routine. Put first things first. Yourself. Also, it's not about being the master of morning routines. Rather, it is about building a foundation and making progress that makes the difference. But don't worry if you already have a good morning routine in place. Let this serve you as a reminder of how powerful a morning routine can be and give me the chance to inspire you to upgrade your routine and make it even more impactful.

It is helpful to remind ourselves that if we do not take care of ourselves first thing in the morning, we often get swept up in our day and are unable to fit our routines in after the morning has passed. Lastly, "winning the day" does not have to mean that we are sky high in the clouds. There will be days that we are barely keeping our heads above the water. So when tough times roll around, we know that we have an anchor that keeps us grounded. Our morning routine is that anchor.

KEY FEATURES OF A MORNING ROUTINE

So let's check out some key features that I have found a powerful morning routine should be. A morning routine should encompass these aspects. It should be essential, effective, sustainable, holistic, versatile and personalized. Let's look at each in turn.

- *It's essential*: Focus on what habits truly make a difference for you in the morning.
- *It's effective:* Our morning routine needs to provide us with the effect that we seek.
- *It's sustainable:* Consistency. Always a must have.
- *It's holistic:* Integrative care for your body, mind and spirit - all in balance.
- *It's versatile*: We need to be able to adjust well towards the situations we find ourselves in every day.
- *It's personalized*: Everyone's rollercoaster ride looks different. So while we can be inspired by others, ultimately, we need to build our own morning routine.

Don't worry, you don't have to memorize this list. I have made sure that these features are implemented in the toolbox to build your own morning routine later on in this chapter.

HABIT BUILDING

I will not ramble about the ins and outs of habit building but will rather leave you with some helpful techniques around which you can build your morning routine. While a morning routine is usually one comprehensive block of time that you can use, which makes it easier to stick to the routine, it might still be helpful to have some techniques at your disposal in case you need them. I recommend skimming this section; you can always get back to it if you need to!

EXAMPLE: A TABATA SET

To illustrate the techniques, I will use the example of doing a tabata set as a habit I would like to build. A tabata set is a 4-minute high intensity workout routine.

- *Habit stacking:* Stack your new habit with an existing one. For instance, I always do my tabata set before I start brewing my coffee in the morning.

- *Trigger is everything*: Have a post it-note on the coffee machine or in the bathroom where you brush your teeth. I have a post with the words "Tabata set" on my coffee maker.

- *Reward yourself:* Experience the good feeling after having completed your habit and integrate a positive statement. I use this statement: "I just love my morning tabata set. Let's go Aaron!"

- *Love the habit*: Ask yourself: "How would this look like if this were fun?" To make my Tabata set fun, I have created a playlist with three of my favorite songs that I use when I do my tabata routine.

- *Make it easy:* Ask yourself: "How would this look like if this were easy?" The answer to this is very individual. Go with what comes to your mind. To make it easy for me, I decided that I would do my tabata directly before my morning coffee.

- *Commit:* An easy way to boost your consistency is just stating where, when and how you will do your habit. I have created this for consistency: "I will do my morning tabata set right before my morning cup of coffee with my favorite songs playing loud!"

- *Environmental design*: Your environment is very influential in your habit building. Create an environment that supports your successful completion of the habit. I asked myself: "What would my environment look like if I was a tabata pro?" I realized that always having my workout gear visible creates a supportive environment for me.

- *Track to keep momentum:* Use a habit tracker if it helps you keep the momentum for doing your habits. I have found that it is a rewarding feeling to check off a box each day when I complete my tabata set.

- *Together is better*: This one is simple. Do your tabata routine with someone. This one is great because of the high likelihood that you will push through even when you sometimes lack motivation.

- *Accountability:* If you cannot do your routine with a friend, commit to them that you will do your routine and report to them every day for two minutes. Set a time for this accountability check in. It can be a voice call or a simple message.
- *Two-minute rule:* This one is not applicable for the tabata set since it's four minutes. But the basic premise of this rule is that consistency is key and that it is best to first build consistency with a two-minute version of the routine. Once you are performing the two-minute version consistently, start adding time and complexity to your routine.
- *Never miss twice*: If you miss once, that is fine. Life happens. But do your best to never miss twice. You generate a negative momentum faster than you think. So please be really diligent about this.
- *Set an alarm:* Set an alarm to do your tabata set.
- *Identity mantra:* Ask yourself: Who is the person who embodies that habit? I repeat this to myself: "I am a tabata pro."
- *Root motivation*: Ask yourself "why?" as often as you need to in order to get to the root motivation of your habit. My reason is answered by this statement: "I want to do tabata to be healthy." Why? "I want to do tabata to feel like a role model to my kids!" A deep "why" can move mountains, my friend.

EXERCISE:
HOW TO CREATE A MORNING
ROUTINE: SETTING THE STAGE

It's game time. Take time right now to do this exercise.

If you are not able to take aside twenty or thirty minutes now, my tip would be to find a time today during which you can do the exercise and set an alarm for that time and come back to the chapter when the alarm rings.

Set up your space so that you are comfortable and make it conducive to reflection. You can take a cup of tea or coffee, play some relaxing music and even light a candle or some incense. Get a journal or your computer so you can jot down your ideas.

Let's get started.

Suggestions for the game: Skim the material in this section first, then dive deeper. Get an overview. Be conscious. Don't blindly follow the steps. Pick and choose what works for you. You want this to be personalized to you to increase your chances of success. Play full out. Have fun.

To start off with, I would like to level out the playing field. You cannot blindly add a new routine if there are other routines or other hurdles holding you back from performing your routine effortlessly. So the first thing that you will do right now is eliminate the things that do not serve you in the morning.

1. In your head, go through your present morning routine in chronological order. Look out for habits and events that you feel a resistance towards or that do not serve to energize your body for the day. Write all these things down.
    a. Looking at your phone, checking emails, scrolling through social media, hitting the snooze button over and over or eating sugary breakfast foods are some things that may not be working for you.
2. Look at your list. Ask yourself why you wrote these things down.
3. Now you are faced with three options. For each of the things on the list, decide what you want to do:
    a. Keep the habit without a change.
    b. Keep the habit but only with some changes that feel good to you.
    c. Throw it out of the window. If you choose to eliminate a morning activity that involves someone else, communicate with the other person and inform them of what you are doing and why you are eliminating the activity.

Congratulations. You now have eliminated resistances in your morning routine and are ready to take the next step.

BUILDING THE FOUNDATION

Let's build the first part of your ideal morning routine: the foundation. Later, we will deal with growing and maintaining your routine.

For the foundation, we are going to brainstorm ideal routines for your morning.

Please make a chart with three columns. The column titles are: body, mind and soul. Breathe. Ask yourself: "What things would I really enjoy doing in the morning? What things really energize me?" Write down all the things that come to your mind. Put them in the proper column. Add the morning routines that you currently do that you have decided to continue to the list. Take as much time as you need.

Next to each activity, write down the amount of time that the routine ideally takes, plus 50% of that time as a buffer. Trust me. Make it easier on yourself by rounding the number upwards.

IMPLEMENTATION

You cannot implement everything on your list. It's impossible. Thus, take the time to highlight about one to three practices of each column that you think are absolutely essential. The following questions should help you make good decisions.

1. Why do I want this?
2. Does it feel like a "*Hell Yes!*" when I think about doing this practice in the morning?
3. Would I be happy to do this every morning for the rest of the year?

Great. You have identified the practices that are likely to make the most difference for you in your morning routine. Now, you have to check in with how much time these practices take and how much time you actually have.

Think about your mornings and decide how many minutes you are truly able to dedicate for your morning routine. Compare with your highlighted practices. See if they match up and if they don't then adjust accordingly until your amount of time available and your chosen practices match.

If you have time left, keep this time unassigned for now, so that it can act as a buffer. If you are in a deficit of time, please cut down even more. Remove practices to make this possible, but make sure to keep at least one practice for each column.

At this point you should have a morning routine in place for your body, mind and soul that also fits your schedule. Make sure that it is truly essential, effective and holistic. The last two things we need to integrate is making it versatile and sustainable.

VERSATILITY AND SUSTAINABILITY

To make the routine versatile, think about the way your morning routine might change on special days. These could include weekend-trips, oversleeping, feeling totally tired, kids needing attention, or anything else that disrupts your plans.

Unforeseen circumstances can happen for anyone, so it is vital to have a safety routine. This is the minimum format of your ideal routine. It is used when you are unable to do your ideal routine. The beauty in this is that you should be able to do your safety routine, no matter what happens. It is your safety net to keep you above the water at any time.

Ask yourself: "How could I cut down my morning routine in case of an emergency?"

Write down your morning safety routine.

Now, the other beautiful thing about the safety routine is that sustainability of your routine is basically pre-built in for you. No matter what happens on a given morning, you will always succeed in doing your routine because you are able to fall back on your safety routine if need arises. This will allow you to feel a sense of accomplishment no matter what happens. This is essential for success.

Have your ideal morning routine and your safety net morning routine written out and openly visible for the next month. It helps greatly.

You did it. Your ideal morning routine plus your safety routine. This foundation should already enable you to keep your head above the water, always and occasionally have your head in the clouds. The baseline should be an elevated state, ready to fly into your day. If you feel like this is not the case, please review and see what is missing to get there.

GROWING THE FOUNDATION

The heavy lifting is done. Now, we will make sure to strengthen your foundation. Add these practices to your foundation if you feel like they help. If not, skip them. Let's jump right in.

1. Growing together: Doing something together is more fun, easy and sustainable. Go ahead if you feel like that is for you and check in whether you and the other person are aligned with what you want to do.
2. Introducing free flow: Less structure, more free flow. What I have found works best is to have your list with all the practices for mind, body and spirit ready and pick one that feels intuitively right from each column in the morning. I highly recommend sticking with a minimum of one practice for each, body, mind and spirit. It will ensure that you will keep your head above the water.
3. Head in the clouds: It would also be awesome to have a practice or two in our toolbox that will move your head closer to the clouds.

The question to ask yourself here is: "What practice can I do in the morning that will enable me to feel like I could move mountains today?" For me, it's a self-pep talk in the mirror with some blasting-loud music on. What's yours?

4. From habits to rituals: A ritual is really something that is speaking to your soul. Ask yourself: "How can I make my habit feel more like a sacred ritual?" E.g. I usually do my weekly review with my favorite festival mix turned up to the max.

5. Design your environment: This one is relatively simple. Ask yourself: "What does the environment look like in which I am most happy to do my morning routine?" Come up with at least three changes you can immediately make to create that environment.

MAINTAINING THE FOUNDATION

It's time to check in and look out for potential roadblocks that could keep you from achieving your morning routine. The same tips from above apply here as well: Skim this section first. Get an overview. Be conscious. Don't blindly follow the steps. Pick and choose. Play full out. Have fun.

1. *Head above the water:* Sometimes, it feels impossible to keep your head above the water. Even the safety routine feels like too much. In this scenario, be super kind to yourself. The only thing I advise here is to just allow yourself to feel what you feel and try to be grateful even now. Gratitude is like the sunlight piercing the night, no matter how dark it seems. I just encourage you to do your best to feel the gratitude swirling in your body.

2. *Reflection:* This is simple. After you have practiced your morning routine for some time, ask yourself: "Do I feel intrinsically rewarded by doing my morning routine?" Adjust if necessary.

3. *The slowest hiker:* Often, there is one routine that you are struggling with more than the others. Ask yourself what you can implement

to increase the success rate of your least accomplished habit. Or ask yourself if this habit is actually necessary in your morning routine. Perhaps this habit fits better somewhere else in your day.

4. *Resistance:* Do you feel resistance towards your morning routine or a part of it? Ask yourself: "Why do I feel this resistance towards (fill in)?" Afterwards, ask yourself: "How can I release this resistance and be in my flow again?" If nothing helps, talk with someone you trust and get to the root issue.

5. *Buffering*: If you feel like your morning routine takes more time than you think, please be honest with yourself about this. It does not help to cram in this important practice. Rather, try to either cut the time of your existing routine by shortening routines or cutting out one. The other option and the one I prefer is to buffer in about 30 minutes for my routine every morning.

6. *Holiday:* What if you have a complete day off or are on holiday? Well, I have tried how it feels not to do my routine versus staying consistent. Surprise, the latter is better. It is mostly based on a mindset that we feel like we do not want to do our morning routine on days off. But we need to realize a hard truth: The day ahead will be significantly more enjoyable when the morning routine is done. Period. Be honest with yourself.

7. *Accountability*: One of the best ways of maintaining your routine is working together with someone you trust. That can range from checking in with someone else on a weekly basis to having a daily call or short message to check in and reflect on your progress. You choose.

So here we are. Morning routine and all. Still in the rollercoaster of life. Slowly making our way forward. What a thrilling ride.

I hope you were able to build or update your morning routine so that you will always be able to keep your head between the surface of the water and the top of the clouds.

In case you found this guide helpful, I would be honored if you would revisit this section of the book whenever you need guidance with your morning routine. What an honor it was to ride with you for this brief time of the chapter. Have fun with the rest of the book. May we meet again.

~Aaron

Wake up determined. Go to bed satisfied.
~ D W A Y N E   J O H N S O N

ABOUT THE AUTHOR

Aaron designs his life to be unconventional and experimental. He loves to ask a lot of questions about life, especially how to live a life of fulfillment in the 21st century. He is using his life as a living experiment in how to have an incredible life.

Aaron started out at university but then he decided to forego a traditional university education in order to brave his own path, trying to find the best way to fill his own time on planet earth.

Currently, Aaron is fascinated with ways to pursue the depths of muscle & strength as an effective tool for lifelong health. He is coaching clients in the 10X strength building modality and his goal is to train 10.000 10Xers around the globe. 10X is probably the shortest and most effective strength training you will find on the planet. In 30 minutes a week, you claim strength, muscle gain, and cardiometabolic health at the same time. For the rest of your life. That is something indeed.

Aaron would love to connect with like-minded souls. So feel free to reach out to him.

Contact Information:
Instagram: @essentialistbody
Website: essentialistbody.com

DEDICATION

I credit the wonderful teachers that I was blessed to learn techniques from. They include Vishen Lakhiani, Jim Kwik, Steven Kootler, James Clear, Greg McKeown, Ronan Diego De Oliveira, Greg McKeown, Steven R. Covey and my wonderful coach, Michael Danklefs.

Through discipline comes freedom.

~Aristotle

CHAPTER 17

DISCIPLINE IS MY COMPASS

by David Priego

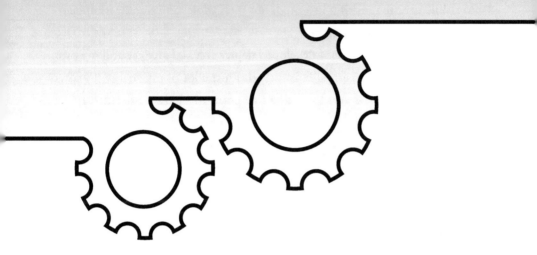

TOPIC:	Creating Healthy Habits
TOOL:	Self Discipline
TECHNIQUE:	Change your mindset so that you can develop the proper mindset to change your current state of health and wellness.

Find what you love to do and go do it.
You will never be successful until you have a plan,
and the discipline and determination
to go through with that plan.

~ J U L I U S   W I L L I A M S

My name is David Priego, I'm from Spain, currently in my forties and I have a lot of experience to share with you on self-discipline, since I'm a professional procrastinator.

Since I was a child I wanted everything to be perfect: to be the perfect kid, excel in my studies, be a great friend. You know the type. I wanted to be great at everything. I was very goal oriented and had great self-discipline to fulfill almost anything I wanted, but then adolescence made its appearance and my whole life changed.

When I was seventeen I developed depression and anxiety and my projections, my perfect-happy-life vanished. I lost a lot of my energy, I wasn't taking care of myself and I was at a low point in my life. I decided that I needed to heal myself, so I went on a journey of discovery. I started learning from the best teacher possible: failure. And also started the most beautiful travel ever, a travel inwards, a travel to know and understand myself.

It took me years to regain my power back and years to regain my health and my ideal weight. Food was my drug. I couldn't resist it.

For years I tried learning tools, techniques, diets, programs and reading articles on the internet. I did it all, but the yo-yo effect always brought me back to where I started. I didn't know how to get out of the cycle.

Things took a downturn in 2018. I had a severe injury on my left calf that had me in recovery mode for almost four months. It was a difficult time for me, but little did I know that this setback would be a trigger that would eventually change the course of my life.

Since I was so tired of Netflix and TV, I bought a pair of airpods and started listening to many podcasts. I dove even deeper into personal transformation and self development and I learned about so many different aspects of health and wellness. I studied nutrition and exercise. I learned about energy and hypnotherapy. I learned about the mind and how to change your mindset. I learned about anything and everything I could so that I could change my circumstances.

Then came the global pandemic. It was March 2020 and Madrid was in full lockdown. I was living alone in a small flat. I had no terrace and no way to get fresh air or exercise. It felt very bleak for me, as it did for many people around the world.

I faced a choice at this point. I could continue developing myself and getting healthy or I could give up and just eat and drink my way through the pandemic. Thankfully, I chose the first path and I am so happy that I did.

I decided to focus on my nutrition by diving deep into why I ate the foods I ate. I got very honest with myself as I examined my eating habits and this helped me to understand that I had always used food in a detrimental fashion. As I said, food had become like a drug for me. I decided to change my mindset and think about food as something that nourished me and helped me to be strong and maintain high energy levels.

Day by day, I built new, healthier habits into my life. I was proud of myself and this helped to increase my self discipline. It was incredible. My mindset had changed and that allowed me to implement what I needed in order to become the healthiest version of myself. I was thrilled with my progress. For the first time in many years, I was feeling energetic and optimistic.

By the time that the lockdown ended three months later, I was a totally different person. I had lost weight, I was looking great, I was happy and most importantly, I had my power back.

Life is not perfect and there are a lot of contingencies along the way.

The years since I first went on my journey have not been easy but through it all, I kept a positive mindset and I continued learning.

In December of 2021 I had an accident and had to recover for a few months, but once I was healed I was right back on track with my habits. I celebrated that.

Then, in the first quarter of 2022 during a regular test doctors told me I required a small surgery in my left kidney. Again I had to stop my training and it felt like I was back to square one. But this time, I knew I would be alright once I recovered from the surgery.

I remember thinking about how the terminator said, "I'll be back." It became my mantra. I repeated this over and over to myself and believed in myself that I could jump right back into my healthy lifestyle soon. I knew that discipline was my compass and I was happy to continue my journey to the best of my abilities no matter what happened. And I did.

Now you might be thinking: "Ok, David, thanks for telling me your story, but how do I implement self-discipline in my own life?"

Below I will summarize some ideas, stories and tips to help you begin the most amazing trip of self-discovery and self-development. Let's go!

SELF DISCIPLINE

At first it takes courage and a lot of energy to focus on yourself. Many times, we want to fulfill the needs of others and please them, but once we've discovered the power of discipline and habits, the world changes.

Discipline is my compass, it marks the way of my heart and helps me achieve my goals. Even after a setback, I need to restart and get momentum.

Discipline is like a muscle and therefore at first you need to learn how to exercise and develop it. The first steps are the most important ones, since you are creating the foundation. Through ownership, reinvent yourself and create the life of your dreams. Self-discipline is a key ingredient to success and as Jim Rohn said, "Discipline is the bridge between goals and accomplishments."

Discipline is also like a ship, a container of habit stacking that serves you to navigate in the sea of life. Depending on the seas you want to sail in, you will continue to need a better, bigger, stronger ship.

Imagine for a moment explorers, like Magallanes and Elcano, who decided to embark on a mission that changed the course of history. They did something that nobody thought possible, trying to find a shorter route for the Silk Road. At the time everybody told them that the world was flat, but they had a different idea. It took a lot of courage and grit, tons of grit, but they believed in their goals, they fought for them and they showed the world they were right. They discovered that the world was round.

Amazing, right? It was faith and discipline which helped them stick with their ideas and ideals so that they could achieve this amazing feat.

Discipline is a way to take action. It is a crucial step in moving forward, in getting yourself to stop thinking and start doing more. Having discipline will help you to achieve better and faster results.

Discipline is doing what needs to be done, when you have to, even if you don't want to do it. Discipline is also a great way to rewrite your inner software, to rewire your brain. Once you install habits that work for you, you realize that you are capable of so much more than you thought and this helps you to expand your comfort zone. You start discarding inherited ideas and beliefs, building a consistency that will give you the outcomes that you truly desire. Discipline helps us to change those stories that disempower us and trade them for stories that empower, motivate and inspire us.

Rafael Nadal, the tennis player, is for me one of the best examples of self-discipline. He deploys a set of rules and habits during his training and while he is playing in tournaments. He is very methodical in his preparation and is always ready for anything. He learns from both success and failure and has a great ability to start again and again. This is one of the amazing trademarks of his and it is also one of the keys for his amazing career and for his incredible comebacks.

Now let's go for some practical stuff. Let's talk about discipline.

DISCIPLINE

Discipline is a word we have all heard, but what is the true meaning of the word discipline? The word "discipline" comes from the latin word disciplina, meaning "teaching and education" and derives from discipulus ("disciple"). Its root word is discere—"to learn".

It usually refers to a coordinated and systematic way of doing things according to a method or code. Discipline helps to learn faster and more efficiently.

Theory is great, but you are reading a book on practical tools and personal experiences that will help you to learn easier and faster, therefore, let's get back to earth. Let's learn some simple steps to develop your discipline.

EIGHT SIMPLE STEPS TO DEVELOPING DISCIPLINE

1. *Acknowledge your weak points*: Nobody is perfect and the first step to change something is to know what to change. Take the time to write down your weak points and think of them as areas that need improvement. Knowledge is power.

2. *Avoid temptations:* Discipline is about doing, it's a habit. If you know that something doesn't help you, try to minimize it or substitute that behavior with another one. If it's complicated for you at first, try breathing before falling into the temptation. Use a pause to take a breath when you want to do something that is not healthy and this might stop you from making that choice. Use the pause for your benefit.

3. *Focus on Your Vision and Make a Plan:* Do you know exactly what you want? How can you achieve it? It's important to have a clear destination. Think of your plan for your life as a sort of global positioning system. With a GPS, you need to introduce a destination in order to find the best route and this is true for your life as well. So create a great vision and then make a plan. Start with baby steps.

4. *Create Sustainable New Habits:* As discipline strengthens you can include new habits. Keep them simple and easy. One new habit at a time.

5. *Health Habits first:* First things first. We need energy in order to feel great so that we can fulfill our daily activities and install our new habits. Start with eating better food, exercising a little more. You need a strong body and will to start, but then these habits will

help to recharge you so you can create new habits. It works as a positive feedback loop.

6. *Practice:* Practice makes perfection. Try Kaizen philosophy by improving just 1% more each day. Cumulative changes make the difference.

7. *Do Not Limit Yourself:* Dream It. Believe It. Create It. Live It. Say bye bye to limiting beliefs because you are limitless.

8. *Reward:* If you succeed, reward yourself. If you fail, forgive yourself. Keep going. As Dory from *Finding Nemo* said… just keep swimming!

It's time for a wrap… Thanks for reading. I really hope my life experience, stories, tips and ideas might have helped you in some way.

Please, do not hesitate to contact me online. I'd love to know about your progress in this amazing journey of self-discipline, a bridge to fulfill your dreams and goals.

Thanks for taking the time to explore your own limits by reading this book. You are awesome. You are extraordinary. Keep evolving, since by doing so you might change your world and therefore The World.

To infinity and beyond!

I send you all of my best wishes,
David

The price of excellence is discipline.
The cost of mediocrity is disappointment.
~ WILLIAM ARTHUR WARD

ABOUT THE AUTHOR

Those who know David well describe him as a "sunny" person, easy going, extroverted, talkative and very curious. His curiosity in fact led him to explore and learn about many apparently unrelated subjects such as Psychology, Cinema, Animation, Photography, Sales and Coaching.

David is a lifelong student and is constantly expanding his knowledge by taking online courses, reading, listening to uplifting content and reading scholarly articles.

David is an avid reader and has devoured books on personal development ever since his teen years. He finds self-actualization and self-improvement fascinating.

Connecting the dots is his passion and with his great communication skills, he plans to become a speaker and content creator as his knowledge expands.

Contact Information:
Email davidpriego@gmail.com
Instagram: @iamdavidpriego

Your body holds deep wisdom.
Trust in it. Learn from it.
Nourish it. Watch your life transform
and be healthy.

~Bella Bleue

**Our bodies are our gardens,
to which our wills are gardeners.**

~William Shakespeare

CHAPTER 18

BODY TALK: HONORING YOUR BODY

by Chanthy Thong

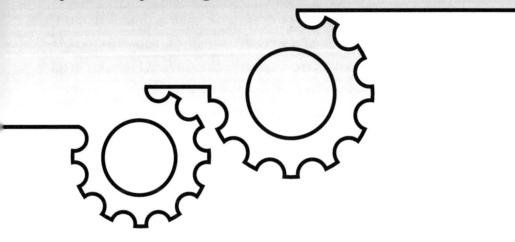

TOOL:	Ayurveda: Body Talk
TOOL:	Body Treatment
TECHNIQUE:	Loving all of your body through all stages of life.

Love yourself first and everything else falls into line.
You really have to love yourself
to get anything done in this world.

~ LUCILLE BALL

My health journey started from the moment when I found out that I was pregnant with my son. Experiencing this little human being growing inside my body amazed me. It was so wonderful and I absolutely loved the journey and welcomed my body to motherhood.

And then my body talk kicked in. On a conscious level, I asked myself, "Have you done enough for this body to be healthy enough for this pregnancy?" A lot of young women think being young, in your twenties, that everything will be fine. They think they have all the time in the world to study, have a career, travel the world, run multiple businesses, become a mother and have it all. In the magazines, billboards and runways in the 1990's and early 2000's, what was considered the ideal body was super thin. Being skinny was in. Skipping your breakfast and running your body on empty was the new normal.

Although this type of diet is not healthy, it is doable for younger people. When you are in your teens or twenties, you can treat your body this way and still be able to function. As you get older, it gets harder and harder. Our body can't handle it. Eating poorly puts stress on the body and it results in a host of problems. The stress is real.

As we move into adulthood, we might have an unhealthy relationship with food. We might eat for comfort or convenience. We might be under lots of stress as we try to find time for everything we need to do. We try to juggle having enough time for sleep, exercise at the gym and preparing healthy foods as we handle all the other aspects of our life like our relationships and family and career. We become super busy with living.

I struggled to maintain the proper life work balance and I tried to deal with all the stresses that came with adulthood. My diet and exercise suffered because I didn't have time for everything and I figured that my body could handle it. I didn't take great care of my body during this time, but I was still able to function.

When I got pregnant, it felt like a miracle. I wanted to do everything I could to make sure my baby was developing properly. I focused on nourishing my body during my pregnancy because I knew it was essential for the baby's health, but also so I could get back into shape after having the baby. It was so important for me to become healthy and have optimal health.

During this time I learned to become kinder with my body. I built awareness around the language I was using about my body. It started with the little step "What I like about myself is…."

This worked really well for me and I developed a really healthy relationship with my body. I credit my pregnancy with helping me to see how important taking care of my body truly was.

Once I had the baby, it didn't take long for me to lose all the baby weight. I went to the gym and it was like starting from the beginning. At first I couldn't even do ten push ups but eventually, as I stuck with it, I was able to do thrifty pullups. This was empowering! I was really motivated and continued working out. Within about six months, I noticed a huge change. I got into such great shape that I realized I had never been so toned and fit before. I started to fall in love with my body all over again and it was the little steps at a time that were the reason for my wins.

As I became healthier, I learned a lot about health. I learned about a concept called the invisible load which is all the stresses we put on our body in this modern world. These stresses affect our adrenaline and increase the production of stress hormones, which has a ripple effect on all the organs and systems in our bodies. This leaves us feeling exhausted and depleted.

One of the stress hormones that can be detrimental is cortisol. Although small amounts of cortisol can be beneficial to our body, large amounts of cortisol can harm the body. Ideal amounts of cortisol can help with regulating inflammation in the body, as it is a powerful anti-inflammatory. It can manage blood glucose levels and support good energy and vitality.

An excess of cortisol, on the other hand, can slow metabolic rates, cause loss of muscle mass, trigger the muscle cells to burn more energy than fat cells, which increases the fat levels. Too much cortisol can also cause elevated blood glucose levels, endocrine problems, poor sleep, a decreased libido and poor gut health. Cortisol can also negatively affect your memory and cause chronic deep fatigue.

Learning about this was a wake-up call for me. I knew I had to control outside stressors in order to stay in peak health. I decided I needed to become more conscious and connected with my body, mind and spirit.

Even though I was in good shape physically, I didn't feel great emotionally at the time. I had no work-life balance. I was overworked in my business and career. For over twenty five years I had worked almost every day without taking a break. I hadn't let myself rest and this put a toll on my body and mind.

I wanted to have another baby and I was having trouble conceiving. My doctor was telling me at the time, "It's very common for a woman your age to be experiencing this." I remember sitting in her clinic room feeling disappointed. I wondered if my difficulties getting pregnant had to do with my physical and emotional state. I kept asking myself, "Where do I go from here?" I knew I had to change my life.

I decided to take action. I got rid of my business and took some time off to go on holiday. I was still feeling stressed, though and I felt a little bit like I was on an emotional roller coaster. I began to look to food for comfort and I started gaining weight. I gained over 65 pounds (30kg) in less than three months. I could barely even recognize myself.

Along the journey,I met an Ayurvedic practitioner who did a pulse reading on me and then helped me understand what was happening inside my bodyShe told me about my constitution and how there were signs of dosha imbalances. This led me on a journey to learn more about Ayurveda and studying these ancient practices have helped me to finally find the balance of physical, mental and emotional health I had been searching for.

I will teach you a little bit about Ayurveda so that you can apply it to your own life.

AYURVEDA

Ayurveda is the science of life, lifespan and longevity. "Ayu" means life and "veda" means science.

Ayurveda is the world's most ancient, scientific holistic health system. It is a complete medical science embodying both therapeutic and preventive strategies for health. In Ayurveda, there are three constitution types, called doshas and it is important to know about your particular doshas to help you to stay in balance, healthy and happy.

DOSHAS

What are the doshas? The word *dosha* means energy. The doshas consist of the five elements we experience around us: earth, water, fire, air and ether (space). These elements come together to create the three Doshas.

Doshas are also known as mind-body types. They are subtle energies that cannot be perceived but that express particular patterns, unique blends of physical, emotional and mental characteristics.

These natural elements are reflected in our bodies. Fire is hot and powerful, like the digestive system. It consists of light, heat, transformation and metabolism. Water is fluid and cool, like our lymphatic system, flow and liquidity. Earth is dense and grounding, like our structure, solidarity and stability. Air is light and moving, like our breath, motion and nourishment. Ether is the vastness that exists inside us when we still our minds, space and container.

There are three dosha types: Vata, Pitta and Kapha. No one has a body that is entirely one dosha, but rather we are a combination of all three doshas.

Ayurveda is a system of regaining our innate dosha balance, so we always treat the dosha that is out of balance in the body.

Understanding my body type was life changing for me. I am a "Pitta Kapha" body type. In understanding what this meant, I learned to love and honor my body more, using food as medicine to eat more consciously, to nourish and balance my body on a cellular level.

Let's learn a little bit about ayurvedic body types.

THE VATA BODY AND MIND

Vata (Air+Ether) I like to call Vata the wind dosha because it's exactly like that: cold, dry, light, rough, subtle and ever-moving.

If you have excess Vata in the body, your body has too much wind or air energy. The body may produce excess gas due to lack of digestive strength. You may suffer from chronic bloating or constipation. Your skin may be dehydrated and hair may be dry and frizzy.

Excess Vata energy in the mind may cause imbalance like a tornado of thoughts. An excess of Vata dosha may cause a person to feel overwhelmed and they may have a hard time turning off the mind. This excessive thinking can cause difficulty falling asleep as well as causing anxiety.

If this sounds like you as a Vata, work on increasing your Pitta (fire) energy. This entails doing things that are warming and stimulating. Focusing on the Kapha (Earth) grounding energies to regain balance is also helpful.

THE PITTA BODY AND MIND

Pitta (Fire + Water) I like to call pita the fire Dosha because it's known for hot, fiery, light, spreading, sour smell, powerful and transformative.

If you have excess Pitta in the body, your body has excess heat.

In Ayurveda the word for the digestive system is the same as the word for fire, agni. Those with excess Pitta have too much heat in their digestion, causing heartburn, hyperacidity and even ulcers. Heat rises, so when that fire tries to make its way out of the body, it can show up on our faces as acne. If you have chronic acne or acidity, then you have a Pitta imbalance.

Pitta will always feel hot and they will have warm hands and feet. They perspire easily when exercising or doing very little movement. Their perspiration may have a sharp odor because their body is trying to detox. A Pitta mind is organized and sharp, but excess Pitta can cause the person to erupt like a hot volcano. Impatience, agitation and anger are all signs of too much pitta in the system. Pitta often becomes "hangry" and angry if their meals are late, making people around them feel just as miserable as they are. You will need to work on increasing your Vata (wind) and Kapha (Earth) energies to regain balance.

THE KAPHA BODY AND MIND

Kapha (Earth+Water) I like to call Kapha the earth dosha because it's exactly like that: grounded, soft, oily, sweet, steady, sticky, soothing, calm and heavy.

Having excess Kapha in the body will make you feel low in energy. It can be hard to get up in the morning to get the body moving. It can also be hard to exercise.

You have a sluggish digestive system and metabolism slows down and may sometimes have mucus build up, like nasal congestion, sore throat, coughs, colds, or infections. You may gain weight and retain water easily, especially if you eat sweets, carbohydrates and dairy. It's important to stimulate your body through your diet to shake out of your Kapha.

Excess Kapha in the system may cause cold hands and feet. An excess can also lead to allergies and thyroid issues. An excess of Kapha energy causes the mind to become slow and sluggish. You may spend a lot of time reminiscing about the past and have a hard time trying new things. You put the needs of others first, which can lead to a lack of self care. If this sounds like you, work on increasing Vita (Air) and Pitta (fire) energy to regain balance.

Below are some basic guidelines to get you started on your Ayurvedic journey. If you find the information in this chapter inter-esting, it will benefit you to go to an Ayurvedic practitioner to have a full assessment.

WHAT WEAKENS DIGESTION

Kapha Factors:

- Overeating
- Eating before the previous meal is completely digested/snacking
- Drinking iced or chilled drinks often (especially before or during meals)
- Eating kaphagenic foods often (cold/heavy/oily/fried)
- Eating a large or heavy meal at night

Vata factors:

- Eating on the run
- Eating irregularly
- Constant physical, emotional or mental stress
- Skipping meals or prolonged fasting
- Frequent traveling (flying/long car journeys)

Pitta factors:

- Eating spicy, pungent, hot, sour foods regularly
- Overuse of alcohol

Other factors:

- Emaciation due to some disease
- Incorrect administration of panchakarma procedures
- Faulty adaptation of place, climate, season

DETOXIFICATION

It's important to do a detoxing program at least twice a year using Ayurvedic herbs to help reset the body and mind. It is really important to have professional advice and work closely with ayurvedic doctors to support your personalized health journey.

FINAL WORDS

I have continued my studies, taking a variety of courses to expand my knowledge. I am studying Ayurveda as well as becoming a certified health coach. I approach health in a holistic manner now and have created healthy habits that help me achieve optimal health. Having a morning and evening routine is essential to maintaining balance. I also pay attention to my nutrition and I eat plenty of fresh, whole vegetables. Adding in a lot of fun activities and having a strength training and cardiovascular training exercise routine is very helpful as well. Finally, practices like meditation, breathwork and other mindfulness practices help to keep me at ease, in flow and filled with energy.

A holistic approach to health is essential to living as healthy as possible. Listening to what your body is telling you is also super important as you move towards your best health. Learning as much as you can about your body and about health is the key to living as healthy as possible for all the days of your life.

It is so important to understand your body's rhythm and maintaining healthy habits can help you respond better to this natural rhythm of your body. Tuning into your body will help you to notice symptoms and conditions like insomnia, sleep loss, problems waking up in the morning, depression or stress. These symptoms are the way that your body tells you that something is wrong and when you notice them early, you can do something about it.

Holistic health and Ayurveda is a doorway to great health. It has been a pathway that has worked for me and it can work for you too. Once you begin to learn about your body and what it needs, you can learn about different holistic health practices that best support your body. Knowing and loving your body through all the stages of life is such a wonderful gift. Loving yourself more and appreciating the body you have helps to honor the unique gifts we have.

I hope that the information in this chapter has given you an interest in Ayurveda and holistic health. Remember you can heal yourself once you become more connected to your body. The journey begins once you tune in and begin to learn what you can do to live on a more conscious health level. Please reach out to me. I love connecting!

~Chanthy

We do not have the right to feel helpless.
We must help ourselves.
After destiny has delivered what it delivers,
we are responsible for our lives.
~ CHERYL STRAYED

ABOUT THE AUTHOR

Chanthy Thong is the founder of Into Wellness. She is a Registered Remedial Massage Therapist, Certified Holobody and Health Dynamics Coach, Qualified Chef, Hairdresser, Beauty Therapist and Aromatherapist.

She has been in the Hair, Beauty and Wellness industry for over 25 years and is passionate about health, clean beauty, great food, women's health and making a big impact.

Her mission is transforming people's health around the world to live their best healthy life. She is currently working on a cookbook and building a health wellness retreat.

Contact Information:
Email: chanthyhbw@gmail.com or info@chanthyintowellness.com
Website: www.intohealthwellness.com, or www.chanthyintowellness.com
LinkedIn: Chanthy Thong
Instagram: chanthyintohbw

You have the power to heal your life
and you need to know that.
We think so often that we are
helpless, but we're not.
We always have the power of our minds.
Claim and consciously use your power.

~Louise L. Hay

CHAPTER 19

ANCESTRAL WISDOM THAT TOOK ME BEYOND HEALING

by Sonal Ladwa Patel

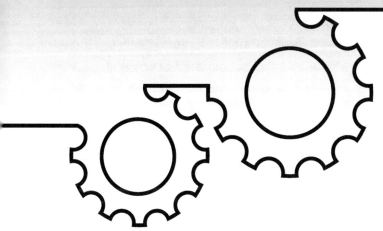

TOPIC:	Healing
TOOL:	Applying Ayurvedic Concept to Self Healing
TECHNIQUE:	Learn more about the ancestral wisdom of Ayurveda. Deeper knowledge of these ancient teachings will help you learn about yourself.

I have lived through much and now I think I have found what is needed for happiness. A quiet secluded life in the country, with the possibility of being useful to people to whom it is easy to do good and who are not accustomed to have it done to them; then work, work of which one hopes to be of use; the rest, nature, books, music, love for one's neighbor- such is my idea of happiness. And then, on top of all that, you for a mate and children perhaps- what more can the heart of a human desire?

~ LEO TOLSTOY

I was fortunate to have had the same realization as Mr. Tolstoy, when I decided to leave the comfort of my home in a bustling city, to find sanctuary in a small rural village in India during the Covid pandemic. Prior to this epiphany I was a stay at home mother of two boys who were born and raised in London, England. Little did I know then that leap into the unknown would help me heal years of poor health and teach me how to thrive in a time when others were trying to merely survive.

After my second child turned one year old our family relocated to Delhi, India. My husband was building his business there and life was busy. I was handling it well and I thought of myself as very resilient. I was not fazed by change and I embraced the international lifestyle, as did our children whom we raised to be resilient to change. We taught our children to seek adventure and to enjoy life.

Five years passed building a life there and although I was able to function well, my health was deteriorating, I started showing signs of inflammatory diseases, including eczema, psoriasis, hair loss and poor digestion. Eventually I developed ulcerative colitis. I could not understand why I was suffering so much. I led what I thought was a healthy lifestyle. I was an active mother of two lively boys and I cooked most of our meals. I made sure to use my culinary skills to create healthy and nutritious meals for the whole family.

Looking back, I realize now that the stresses of unpredictability in our lives living overseas and often with financial difficulties were causing me stress. Loneliness also took its toll as I lost my sense of belonging without my family and friends in England. I became rather reclusive and even though I tried my best to keep upbeat, I lived with a scarcity mindset and I lived in survival mode.

I harbored feelings of anger and resentment, for I had lost my sense of self and purpose. I was too busy being busy as I took care of everyone else. I had depleted my reserves caring for others and never gave a thought to my own self-care. I was a toxic mess inside, which was manifesting on the outside.

From my experience of not only my own health but those of people I have coached, I believe that our mental and emotional state can lead to a host of inflammatory diseases. Poor environment and unhealthy lifestyle choices only escalate the symptoms. In Ayurveda it is believed that disease stems from poor digestion. Everything we take in, from our food, to the air we breathe, any visual stimulation, even our emotions and thoughts are all absorbed through digestion and put strain on our body's digestive function. We are often overloaded with toxins that are not removed effectively.

I tried prescribed medication and ointments to relieve my various ailments, only to find that none of them worked for long. It would heal, but a few weeks later flare up again. I found myself in a vicious cycle of frustration as my self-esteem diminished along with my appearance.

I finally came to the point where I had to figure out how to resolve these issues once and for all. I went on a journey of learning all about health and wellness. I learned that my problem was that I was neglecting my self-care. Although I thought I ate well, my gut function was poor and I was not absorbing as many nutrients as I needed. I also had many intolerances to foods and I was not properly hydrated. I had never struggled with weight but after giving birth to two kids, my body needed some work to become stronger.

I also learned about the mind-body connection and began to understand how the toxic emotions I suppressed affected me. My internal state, my emotional and spiritual state meant that my health would be affected. The body has a remarkable way of healing itself given the right conditions. This was something that I had always firmly believed, but hadn't been able to apply in my life. I was determined to learn how to do this and how to figure out what those conditions were for my own body to heal. I began to look inward to heal what I was experiencing on the outside. I started using the ancestral wisdom I accrued over the years of studying the ancient scriptures including the Bhagavad Gita, Charaka Samhita and other Hindu Vedas.

But one lesson improved my well-being above all others and is still relevant now. I want to introduce you to the three gunas, or attributes of nature. Don't worry if this is your first time learning about them, Just take in what you can and if you find the information applicable to your life, you can learn more about it by buying books on the subject or finding a practitioner in your area.

THE THREE 'GUNAS' (ATTRIBUTES) OF NATURE

With just this one powerful pearl of wisdom, I transformed not only my own state of mind, body and soul, but that of my clients too.

Once you understand the Gunas and how they relate to the mind, emotions and your daily life, you will create awareness around your thoughts and actions. This awareness will help you to transform your life.

The gunas can be thought of as a lens to view yourself. Understanding the gunas will help you to navigate your inner world, which ultimately will affect your outer experience in the world. The Gunas are a part of everything in the universe, but that is for another book. For now, let's focus on how it shows up in our daily lives.

THE 3 'GUNAS' IN THE PHYSIOLOGICAL ASPECT AND OUR EMOTIONAL STATES

Tamas

Experienced as inertia, darkness, obstruction, inactivity, heaviness, stagnation and fear. Tamasic states include laziness, doubt, sadness, hurt, shame, boredom, apathy and ignorance.

Rajas

Experienced as movement, activity, agitation and desire. Rajasic states include passion, alertness, determination, self-centeredness, anxiety, restlessness, anger, greed and worry.

Sattva

Sattva means 'pure essence'. Sattva promotes harmonious, clear, peaceful states. It is experienced as stillness, balance, harmony and clarity. Emotional states include happiness, joy, peace, love, freedom, friendliness, openness, creativity, fulfillment and inspiration.

The gunas are not separate and are in fact intertwined. We can feel elements of all these states separately or in differing proportions at the same time, which makes transition to another state easier.

You can't just move from one state to another without using the various states. For instance, you can't jump to Sattva from Tamas without the leverage that comes from Rajas. Stepping out of stagnation requires action whether you are depressed, overweight or just bored. Positive Rajas movement is what you require to reach a happier place, a feeling of Sattva.

HOW UNDERSTANDING THE GUNAS HELPED ME

Once I learned about these states, I realized I was stagnant in my life. I needed to create movement to become more motivated to find joy and purpose again.

My inner work included reading and educating myself and finding who I was, what I loved and how I wanted to show up in the world. My journey of self discovery led me to become a holistic health coach. I created awareness around my states of being and learned how I could change them to be more positive. It was this mindset that helped me create a life where I found purpose, mental well-being, optimal health and an abundance mindset.

Taking action is the key element,, even if you have to take action that you don't feel motivated to take. The key is to get going and even a baby step in the right direactyion will have a huge impact further down the line. . If you are stuck and not sure how to lift your mood, a forced action or habit can help transform your emotions even if Tamasic. For example, if you are feeling low, you can force yourself to go for a walk outdoors.

Maybe you will choose to smile at anyone who passes by. This will change your emotional state to a more joyful one. Your brain receives the message from your facial muscles and dopamine that is released through exercise will lift your mood. Also, when people smile back you will find a real reason to smile. So the action of taking a walk, even if you don't feel like it, can have a beneficial effect on your physical, emotional and mental state.

With even this basic understanding of the gunas you can use this information to learn about yourself.

You have a tool to look for their manifestation both inside and outside of yourself.

TOOLS

1. We can manipulate the presence of Gunas within ourselves and others by noticing what we choose to pay attention to and what we are consuming (our attention) as well as by choosing how we act (our intention).

2. For each challenge you face in life, ask these questions:
    a. Why am I doing this?
    b. How am I doing this?
    c. What action can I take to move in a positive direction towards a state of Sattva?

3. To optimize your health and well-being, aim to create more Sattva and positive aspects of Rajas.

4. Understand the intention behind an emotion by asking the above questions and then notice how your emotion is being expressed. This will determine if your emotion is predominantly Tamas, Rajas or Sattva in nature.

5. You can then use this as a lens to view possible outcomes more aligned with the Sattva mode.

6. Journal your thoughts and then pinpoint which Guna applied to help create awareness of how they show up in daily life.

HOW TO APPLY THE THREE GUNAS TO DAILY HABITS.

Transform Tamas

1. *Change your sitting position:* The ultimate comfort zone in the West is the couch and it could be slowly killing you! Slouching on the sofa contributes to digestive issues, obesity, back ache and lower libido. I corrected a recurring sciatica issue and my digestion with a few changes to how I sat.

2. *Avoid processed foods*: Eating foods that lower resistance to disease and have a negative impact on the mind are considered Tamasic in nature. These foods are heavy and block flow as they add to toxic buildup 'Ama'. Highly processed foods, alcohol, meat, refined sugars and tobacco are some examples.

3. *Create Awareness:* It is important to become aware of your Tamasic emotional states and then use tools to move into a positive state. Limit your exposure to toxic people and gossip. Instead find a tribe that uplifts you.

4. *Declutter your home:* Decluttering is great for clarity of mind and body. Keep items that are essential or bring you joy. Clean your kitchen of toxic cookware such as aluminum, non-stick coatings and plastics. Replace them with health promoting or neutral cookware like cast iron, stainless steel, copper, earthenware and glass.

5. *Align yourself with the Circadian Rhythm*: Aligning your body clock to the Sun is how you stay in sync and keep your sleep patterns, digestion and hormonal balance optimal. I got used to waking at 5am with help from Robin Sharma's book 5am club, however I realized people in the village already knew these benefits.

Balance Rajas

Create action and movement in a balanced way to move into a positive state. Keep your body moving throughout the day versus an hour in the gym. If you are a stay at home mum like me then get on your hands and knees and give the floor a good old scrub, clean the windows, gardening, walk to get groceries because you'll only buy what you can carry, which means only the necessities will come into your home. Find a reason to move and stay active throughout your day.

1. *Rajasic foods:* These have have a stimulant effect and often provoke mental restlessness. They are not completely beneficial, nor are they harmful to the body or mind. Food that is too spicy, too pungent, too sour or too bitter. Foods and drinks that lift your energy and give you a buzz are also Rajasic in nature.

2. *Sun Salutations: Surya Namaskar:* Traditionally practiced at sunrise for optimal benefits of energy flow that will stay with you throughout the day. This one yoga sequence done daily can improve cardiovascular conditioning, prevent fatigue, promote calm and relaxation, lengthen and strengthen the muscles, aid digestion, increase weight loss and provide a range of other mental and physical benefits. Form is more important than the number of rounds so start slowly and increase rounds daily. This will balance all three Gunas in body and mind with practice.

3. *Grounding:* In nature just as the Gunas that exist in everything we are also made of the same matter and need to connect to feel balanced. Grounding is basically standing or walking barefoot on the Earth, also known as earthing. It helps realign your energy by reconnecting you to the Earth's natural healing energy. Practice barefoot standing or lying on the ground outdoors or even submerged in a water body. It has the power to reduce inflammation, pain and stress; improve blood flow, sleep and vitality.

Develop Sattva

In order to move into a more balanced state, you can use the tools below to develop sattva.

1. *Pranayama*: Make every breath count. The most valuable lesson to get to a Sattvic state is to breathe correctly. Daily conscious practice of breath work can be calming, energizing and even help with stress-related health problems ranging from panic attacks to digestive disorders. "Patanjali in his Yoga Sutras well-being recommends various breathing techniques that involve inhaling, exhaling and breath retention for longevity; these are called Pranayama (vital force). Nasal breathing retention of breath as well is the key for brain optimization.

2. *Eat Sattvic Foods:* In Ayurveda Sattvic foods and eating habits are pure, essential, clean and conscious. Optimal health requires optimal nutrition to feed our mind, body and gut bacteria. The main reason for poor health is poor feeding. Sometimes over feeding!

3. *Fasting:* Fasting is a Sattvic act that purifies the body and mind to bring one closer to enlightenment. Just ask the great Yogi's and Monks who can abstain for days on end. The mind becomes more powerful through abstinence. When I fasted, my clarity of mind and willpower was urging me to go beyond the four days. I had to eat again. The intestine is the most highly regenerative organ in the human body, regenerating its lining every five to seven days. When our digestive system is given a break, the body can focus energy on repair rather than digestion. This is especially important if you are suffering from any autoimmune or inflammation issues as these problems often stem from a permeated gut lining or 'leaky gut'.

PURPOSE (DHARMA)

Life purpose is that burning desire you have inside to do something great. That gut feeling inside that you have found your calling. A little hint, it will generally be something that helps others.

Purpose can also be seasonal and can change as you evolve; it is not always rigid. Turn your ambitions into something that will serve others. This is where you will find the most satisfaction, joy and drive to achieve your legacy. After all, what are we here for if not to leave our mark and be remembered by future generations. If you haven't discovered your life's purpose yet, don't beat yourself up. The more awareness you create around yourself and the three 'Gunas', the clearer it will become. Embrace the learning curve and remember that you are on a lifelong journey of growth.

HOW DISCOVERING THE GUNAS HELPED ME

During the pandemic I felt the urge to drop into fear pulling at me, but I stood strong and decided I was not going to let my family live like that. Of course I wanted them to be safe but I didn't want them to live in fear and isolation. I wanted them to be free and healthy (Sattva). The only place we could think of to do this as things begin to close down around us was my husband's ancestral home in a small rural village in Gujarat, India. At the time my husband was in Mumbai on his way to Gujarat to meet us. I took my two children and two suitcases of essentials and got us on one of the last flights out of Delhi (Rajas). At the time my husband was in Mumbai on his way to Gujarat to meet us. Little did we know when we made the decision that my husband would contract the virus and be hospitalized and we would not see him when we landed.

This was the first wave and no one knew how to handle it, not even the doctors, there was no protocol or vaccine. We were uncertain he would even come back to us as we began to hear about more and more people dying (Tamas). I knew I had to remain positive for the boys and help them adjust to this new way of life (Sattva). I thought we would only be there for a month but it turned into nine as all flights were grounded.

We turned up at the 1940's house that was in serious disrepair. Termites had eaten their way through the rafters and the ceiling was barely holding up. There was dust on everything (Tamas). I kicked into action to get the house back to a livable state (Rajas). The village community were very welcoming and brought us vegetables, milk and grains from their farms. I realized I was not alone and that was a huge relief (Sattva). Even through lockdowns the village was self-sustaining, providing us with everything we needed. It was a comfort that food was not going to be a scarcity. The bonus being it was local, fresh and organic too (Sattva). We soon realized that our small bubble in the village was a safe haven and I felt a sense of belonging after so long without that feeling.

My children experienced freedom they would never have had in the city, playing safely from dawn until dusk with the local kids in nature (Sattva). This was what I wanted for them and it was why I took the leap (Rajas), to not only survive but to thrive.

During this time, we lived on basic rations and simple amenities. To give you an idea, the electricity was a small gas cylinder stove, running water was available but there was no hot water, the beds were rudimentary. The one luxury was a television which was so old my eldest asked, "Mom, what is that on the back of the TV?" To which I replied, "That is the rest of the TV". We had the bare minimum, but it was sufficient and we began to find joy in the simple things.

We spent most of our days outdoors in the courtyard where I would prepare ingredients for meals, wash dishes and do the laundry by hand. We danced in the monsoon rains and walked barefoot in the fields. My husband returned to us three months later a shell of his former self. I made it my mission to heal myself and to help my family thrive. It didn't take doctors or pharmaceuticals. It took going back to basics and living the simple life.

I was big on anti-aging and even began writing articles for an online biohacking magazine. I realized that everything I had been reading and researching was a modern take on ancestral teachings, many from India. So, I decided to test out some of these hacks on a budget and from what I could source in the surrounding village. Turns out this place was abundant in tools for well-being. You won't need to move to a remote village to learn the lessons I am about to share, though I highly recommend it. Let me share some of the practical things that will translate over into your daily life.

As a farming community they are completely in sync with the circadian rhythm. They rise just before sunrise and perform Surya Namaskar (Sun Salutation), not the yoga sequence, but actual offering of prayer and gratitude to the sun upon rising. They bask in the early morning rays for ten minutes or more getting a dose of Vitamin D.

Their meals are also aligned, breakfast is wholesome yet light as it is only to break the fast. In the mornings, digestion is just awakening like the Sun so eating light is best.

Most of their day is outdoors working, except around midday when the Sun is strongest, as is the digestive fire (Agni). This is when they eat their largest meal. After lunch, a short siesta allows the meal to digest, brings focus and energy back so they can go back to work until sunset.

As the sun dwindles so does digestion, therefore the last meal is light, wholesome and easy to digest and it is taken at least three hours before bed. The exposure to blue light from screens is Rajas and prevents a restful sleep. Instead they sit under the Moonlight engaging with family and friends. An early start means going to bed around 10pm. The optimal time for deep restorative sleep is two hours either side of midnight, so try and get all four hours for maximum benefit.

Modern studies are showing that cold water therapy may boost cognitive health. Whether the villagers here knew the benefits or not, they have always bathed in cold water first thing every morning. They also bathe in the evening before having dinner to kick start the digestive fire (Agni).

At first it was a shock to the system, especially in cooler months, but that is the whole point. That shock to the system releases the pain suppressing hormones beta-endorphin and noradrenaline, which help with depression. The surge of these hormones also increases blood flow and clear thinking as well as decreases inflammation. I noticed my skin and hair improved greatly with this practice. The most interesting part was that my family commented on the improvement of my energy levels and mood. I was now more alert, had less brain fog and my memory was better than before.

In the village it is customary to sit on the floor and even meals are eaten in a folded leg position called lotus pose. This pose is good for posture and is optimal for digestion too, as it directs the flow of energy to the digestive organs. Many people squat as their regular means of sitting and even elderly people are able to hold a comfortable full squat for hours. This is fantastic for optimal mobility and longevity.

FINAL WORDS

I hope you have enjoyed learning how ancient practices can help you to live a healthier life. It is my mission to share these teachings with as many people as I can. I am amazed at my own transformation and I want to help others to have their own health transformation. Isn't it incredible that we can completely overhaul everything about ourselves if we put our mind to it?

I wish you luck on your health journey. Please reach out if you want to connect. I would love to hear about your journey.

Best Wishes,
Sonal

Stop looking for happiness in the same place you lost it.

~ PAULO COELHO

ABOUT THE AUTHOR

Transformational Life Coach

Sonal Laswa Patel is an entrepreneur, an author, a public speaker, a house-wife and stay at home mom. She is also an amazing chef and has made appearances on MasterChef UK.

A former fashion designer, actress and model who went from living in London and New York to a small village in India during the Covid pandemic, she transformed her life and discovered her higher calling.

Sonal is on the expert panel for health optimization magazines: Biohackers Update and Time Verse where she shares her knowledge of ancestral wisdom, nutrition and well being.

Beyond these accomplishments, Sonal is mindset mentor, leadership and life coach to celebrities and changemakers across the world.

Her mission is to share life transforming lessons and to coach the ordinary to live extraordinary life.

Contact Information:
UK & Worldwide
sonal.ladwa@gmail.com

PART 4
LIFESTYLE CHOICES: INNER WORLD

I learned that the interior of life was as rewarding
as the exterior of life and that my richest
moments occurred when I was absolutely still.

~RICHARD BODE

PART 4: LIFESTYLE CHOICES: INNER WORLD

Total Health is a way of approaching your life in a holistic manner. We have discussed mindset and the importance of keeping your mind in a positive thinking pattern. Then we turned to the physical aspect of health, which most of us are familiar with. This is where we talked about the importance of nutrition and exercise. We also learned about the daily habits we could install to help us move easily in the direction of vibrant health and wellness.

Now we turn to your inner world.

When you change your inner world, your outer world changes as well. Indeed, everything is first created in your mind and then in the world. Everything you see around you was first thought of in somebody's mind before it was created in the world. This is how all things are created. Changing your inner landscape and creating a space where you feel peaceful and calm will allow you to achieve a healthy emotional state Since the body, mind and emotional state all contribute to your state of health, it's imperative to address all areas in a holistic manner in order to create the healthiest version of you.

The upcoming chapters focus on practices that enhance your inner world. You will learn about visualization practices, gratitude practice and a beautiful practice called 10 Minutes of Joy that will help you to maintain your equanimity regardless of what is happening around you. You will go deep into self inquiry as well as begin to incorporate the age old practice of meditation into your life. These amazing techniques will change your inner state, which will in turn change your outer state.

It's time to get healthy from the inside out.

Being challenged in life is inevitable, being defeated is optional.

~Roger Crawford

CHAPTER 20
OBSTACLES MAKE ME STRONGER

by Nolan Pillay

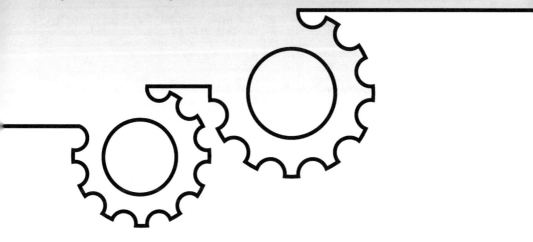

TOPIC:	Visualization
TOOL:	The Silva Ultramind 3 Scenes Technique
TECHNIQUE:	Visualize three scenes. Visualize where you are now, the path to success and then where you want to go.

I have learnt that the obstacle is temporary, use
it as an opportunity to learn and grow.

~ N O L A N P I L L A Y

My life has included many obstacles that I have had to face, but here I am five decades later, standing stronger than ever, feeling healthier and have gained a new understanding of my body and how I should treat it. Let's be honest here, if we don't treat our bodies well, will it serve us long term? The answer is clear… absolutely not!

How did I get through these obstacles you may ask? It's simple, I refused to play the victim or use a self-pity mindset, I made the decision in my head to become the best version of myself and to focus on my body and mind.

Let me share my journey with you…

Growing up in Apartheid South Africa robbed my family and I of many privileges, because we had to live in race segregated areas with poor living conditions. This forced my parents to do basic jobs to put food on the table and clothe us. I recall going to school on a cold, rainy day with no shoes or jersey, feeling the cold biting into my bones. It was the kind of weather that will allow you to get sick easily, but these conditions actually strengthened me.

I could have seen this as an obstacle and stayed away from school, but I knew education was important and the nice part was that the school provided sandwiches for us when we did not have any. Take a few minutes and imagine living a life like this, in extreme poverty, in harsh conditions that no human should experience. That was my childhood.

The beauty from this experience were the values and compassion that helped grow me into the man that I am today. Life's lessons are best learnt when you get to experience them and I certainly learned a lot of life's lessons during my formative years. The main lesson was to never give up. Giving up was never an option for us.

There were moments of joy though, as in all lives when we look. I went through a beautiful chapter of my life when I excelled in sports. You name it, I was good at it. So good that I was named sportsman of the year for five years running. I knew I could have been a professional in sports but again, the apartheid system took that away from me. The system prevented a person of color from representing their country, irrespective of my talent. I strongly believed that I had the capabilities to excel in sports, but was not able due to the political situation in my country at that time. I will say that it didn't stop me from playing though. I continued to be active because I loved how it made me feel confident and how it kept my body in shape.

Another huge obstacle I had to grapple with in my life was depression when I was younger. Depression, something that affects us all at some point in our lives, is not an easy thing to deal with unless we learn some techniques to overcome it. For me, my depressive state came about when I failed my matric exam and tried to commit suicide. This was the lowest I actually felt as a person. I know, you might say that surely it could not have been that bad. And looking back, it wasn't that bad, but when you are in that state you don't always see the light at the end of the tunnel. Things seem dark. If I could go back to my younger self, I would go back and say, "Don't be stupid, life is not that bad." But alas, we cannot go back. We can only go forward.

But you see when you are young, experiencing every obstacle possible, you are inexperienced and you have no idea how to deal with it. You may have moments when suicide becomes the only way out. This period of my life was hugely difficult for me. Back then, my focus was on what people thought about me, what the community would say about me and how my family would feel about me. I wondered, would they call me a failure? The embarrassment alone drove me to do things that I would never have imagined.

It was a traumatic time in my life, but it was also a period of time that shaped me and created the foundation for the person I would become. I look back at this episode of my life now and smile and feel grateful and thankful that I survived to tell the tale. If I had not, I would not be writing this chapter to you and expressing my life stories.

When I connect the dots of my life, I come to realize that no matter what I went through, it was all part of my life's journey. Without these fundamental obstacles as lessons, I cannot imagine how my life would have played out.

I have learned that it's important to find the gifts in your situation because there are always gifts. For instance, I am very appreciative of the things I have now, things like clothes on my body and food in my kitchen. It was the fact that I had been so deprived as a child that made me appreciate the smallest things as an adult. I often wonder how I would have turned out if I was some rich child. Would I be appreciative of the things I have now? I think not!

There are always gifts, as long as we look for them. The key is to change what we focus on. We tend to focus on the things we didn't have rather than the gifts that came from what we did have. Changing your mindset in this small way to look for the silver lining in every cloud is the very first step in creating lasting transformation in life.

So, when I think about and talk about all these obstacles, I realize they made me stronger. I am speaking from my heart about my lived experiences. I spend my life now inspiring others with my life lessons and life stories in the hopes that through my experiences, people will begin to see their own life from a different perspective. So all of the things I went through were necessary for me to be who I am today. For me to be able to help others in similar situations.

I smile even more when I realize that this has been part of God's plan, I was being tested, my strength and courage was being tested.

How strong is Nolan, really? Can he bounce back from this and go further to turn his dreams into reality?

How powerful is it that in our lives, we are put through the most extreme tests to see how we can handle them.

Is this all part of the journey to make us into these humans that can handle anything that is thrown our way? Deep questions indeed that need to be asked, the answers are always revealed in the way our lives are manifesting.

After all the ups and downs, the highs and lows, I have learned one simple thing. I had all the answers within me the entire time! All of my searching and it turned out that my treasure was right here within me,

I want to take you back to January 2021 as this was almost the end of my journey through life. The world was in lockdown, we were besieged with uncertainty and fear. And then, I was diagnosed with COVID.

I remember thinking, "How did this happen to me? Why did this happen to me? Why is God and the World being unfair to me? Why… Why…Why?"

There I was, back to feeling sorry for myself and living as a victim, self-pity at its highest level. This is how life goes, we go up, we go down. We constantly have to go back and keep learning the lessons until we really understand them. Until they stick. I am only human, experiencing human emotions.

I remember the day clearly. It was a Friday, 16 days after having been diagnosed with COVID-19 pneumonia. I broke down and was in a bad state as thoughts ran through my head.

"Is this the end of my precious life?"

What is going on—people around me are dying? Must I witness all of this and still focus on my recovery? Forward wind, covid struck and put me totally out of my zone. I did not know what was happening to my body but knew this was a stranger attacking my body. I can tell you that this was not an easy journey, but I now call it my new lease on life. I was there to learn that my *WEALTH is MY HEALTH!*

How did I get through 13 days in the Intensive Care Unit?

I had learnt a technique called the Silva Method Three Scenes Technique that I decided to use while I was in the hospital. At my lowest, when I was lying in the hospital bed thinking I might die, this technique popped into my head. So I decided to try it even though I wasn't even really sure if it would work. I began to daily, four times a day and I am sure this is what saved my life.

This is the technique that I used and it's one I want to share with you. You can use it for anything in your life that you want to accomplish, anything that you want to manifest. Here is the way I did it.

THE SILVA ULTRAMIND METHOD

Scene 1: Visualize Where You are Now

In the first scene, I see a mental screen in front of me and portray the pain I am going through. There is no need to dramatize it more as I am experiencing this first-hand. I imagine how this COVID-19 pneumonia has set me back in a bigway, how my confidence has been blown away and what it is doing to my body, which was very well toned before this. How can this be happening to me at my age?

I play the scene out repeatedly with more questioning as to why me. Is this a test of my mind and resilience? I am hurting a lot trying to figure this out. Till now I don't know how I got this dreaded disease, who passed it onto me. Could it have been the chemicals I tasted on my lips when I first noticed my pain and fever? I keep playing this first scene out in my head and make it much worse, to the point that they have now put me on a ventilator. Remember, this meditation is more a visualization technique so keep reading.

Scene 2: Visualize The Path to Success

In the second scene, I play out what I am going to do from my side to help with my recovery. I see the doctors and modern medicine playing their role, the nurses are doing their best and it's also in my interest to play my part and trust the process.

The high-flowing oxygen is also playing its part as it is my lifeline. At this stage, I am doing my daily practices like gratitude, meditation, positive self-talk, listening to my mantras, listening to the various religious music and prayers that I am receiving daily... I am playing my part. I take the high dose of pills they give me daily; a lot are vitamins as there is no cure for COVID-19 pneumonia. They help me sleep and this gives me a little energy.

Scene 3: See the Result You Want As if is Achieved

The third and final scene, I now play out that I am well, fully recovered, at home and enjoying being myself again. I go as far as visualizing myself playing in the yard with my grandchildren. I am fit and healthy, doing daily walks with my wife around the dam, just enjoying the peacefulness of nature. When I look around, all I see is an abundance of everything we need. We do not have a shortage of anything.

I imagine talking to thousands of people and sharing my inspirational COVID-19 pneumonia journey with them in the belief that my story and guidance will help save many more lives. People who were living in fear are now saying that if they get COVID-19, they will deal with it. Back to my third scene: I am living blissfully, pain free, my lungs have cleared, I am able to jog and cycle, plus hike again. Everything I loved doing is back as part of my life and this excites me even more.

This is another obstacle I had to face in life and the more I get through them, the more I realize that my purpose on earth still needs to be fulfilled. If you lost a loved one through covid and would like to know what they experienced, you should check out my book called *My COVID Journey* on Amazon, it will help you reach closure and find some peace to move on. I also share some mind hacks and techniques that I used on myself to get through this phase of life.

Earlier in this chapter, I spoke about my suicide episode and now my covid experience. On the one hand I am trying to kill myself and the second, I was fighting to live.

How strange is life that it tests us in this way?

Hang onto your seats, the year started off with covid and it ended on a high with me having to experience a mild heart attack. Can my life get any better? Of course it can and it will.

I got admitted in December 2021 again to the same hospital but this time, the covid experience had caused some damage to my arteries. Eventually, I had three stents put in and was discharged. Was I disappointed at this new development? Yes, this meant I would be on medication, something I am not in favor of, as I don't like putting toxins in my body. Another obstacle endured and I had to move forward stronger than ever.

Guess what, I have realized the power of my body and mind and did the unthinkable in August of this year, I decided to climb Mount Kilimanjaro again, this time it was for a phenomenal cause of giving the gift of hearing to a child and bridging the gap by uniting the Deaf and Hearing communities. Mission accomplished and I am feeling stronger than ever.

Ask me now, how I have learnt to overcome obstacles in life and use them as motivation to make me stronger?

Obstacles Make Me Stronger is now on Udemy for you to learn more about who Nolan is and his journey through Life.

Feel free to connect with me. Much Love and Light.
Nolan

ABOUT THE AUTHOR

Nolan Pillay is a Human Mindset Specialist, a Life Coach, Inspirational and Motivational Speaker, Enlightened Warrior and Author of his latest book *My COVID Journey.* He is also the brilliant and dynamic founder of the trademarked self-development program: Be the BEST Version of YOURSELF™ running under the company StraightTalkWithNolan (Pty) Ltd. His latest online course called *Obstacles Make Me Stronger* speaks about mental wellness, depression, suicide, limiting beliefs and how we as humans go through life allowing ourselves to feel suffocated can be found on Udemy.

Nolan is also Philanthropist, together with his foundation *Be the BEST version of YOURSELF* work on various projects. This year they climbed one of the highest mountains in Africa, Mt Kilimanjaro to raise funds and give the gift of hearing to a child. Even more inspiring is that five of the seven climbers are from the Deaf community, he believes this is the start to bridge the gap between the Hearing and Deaf communities.

Contact Information:
Author's email nolan@straighttalkwithnolan.com
Instagram - https://nolanpillay360.com/

Calmness of mind is one of the beautiful jewels of wisdom.

~James Allen

CHAPTER 21
MEDITATION IS A LIFESTYLE
by Claudia Valentinuzzi Núñez

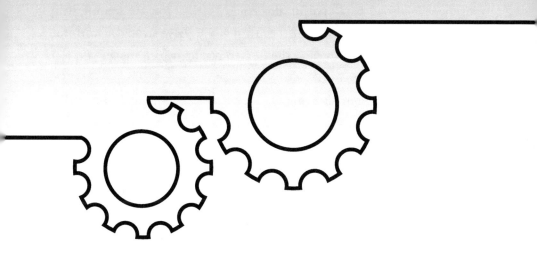

TOPIC:	Stress Relief
TOOL:	Meditation
TECHNIQUE:	Add meditation into your life by starting with a short meditation. Start small and build your meditation practice from there.

When meditation is mastered, the mind is unwavering like the flame of a candle in a windless place.

~ BHAGAVAD GITA

If you are reading this book, you are probably looking for help to overcome a major health challenge in your life.

Health challenges can happen in various ways. It could be an unexpected situation that changes your life suddenly and makes you feel scared and worried. Or it could be a situation you expected, but still, knowing that it became real and finally having to face it, makes you feel overwhelmed and paralyzed. It also could be that you are seeking help to improve some aspect of your health that you have struggled with for a long time, without achieving the desired results, which makes you feel frustrated and disappointed.

Regardless of your situation, you have probably decided to buy this book because you want to find solutions. This is great. Take a moment now to acknowledge yourself for taking the steps you need to create a healthier lifestyle.

Before we get going, let me mention that you may find an extra obstacle along the way that you should consider. Whenever you decide to begin a journey and you have to decide a direction to go in, be aware that you should not put pressure on yourself. Remember that change takes time, so remove any feelings of having to take immediate action and simply allow yourself to be in an information gathering mode right now. You want to avoid putting added pressure on yourself right now so you don't drop into an even more intense whirlpool of negative emotions where you end up feeling even more worried, overwhelmed and frustrated.

Allow this book to educate you, inspire you and empower you to take action. Remember, the mission is to recover your health, so be patient and kind to yourself during the process. Trust yourself.

As you begin your journey towards health, you will be looking deep within to learn more about yourself. This will allow you to find the root cause of the health situation you are currently in. Along the way, you may have to face some painful truths you have been avoiding but remember, the only way to truly heal is to find the root cause and work to heal from there. As you deal with these deeper issues, you will find an inner strength that you didn't even know existed. You will learn to stop doubting yourself and that is when you will find the strength you need to fight for your health.

If along the way your biggest problem becomes you do not trust your own inner strength to do what is necessary to fight for your health, let me tell you that you are not alone. There are many of us who doubt our strength. Many of us doubt we can do what is necessary. Personally, I know what it feels like to believe that I cannot make it. I know what it feels like to fail repeatedly. Along the way, though, I learned how to overcome my doubts and conquer my inner strength and I want to share my story because maybe it will help you.

When I was younger I was obese, but I overcame it in my twenties. I did this by adopting a healthy lifestyle, with very good eating, exercise and rest habits. I was in good health. I was a successful professional and my personal life was great as well.

In my thirties, my health began to deteriorate and I learned I had a thyroid disorder. At this point, I began to put on a few pounds which upset me greatly. I became obsessed with losing these extra pounds, but no amount of effort seemed to work.

In addition, the thyroid disease caused me terrible mood swings and I began to suffer from depression. The combination of my weight losing obsession and my depression gradually led me to also suffer from anxiety and bulimia. This lasted for ten years and they were very difficult for me as I faced intense depression, which seemed to get worse over time. As my depression worsened, my health situation became dramatically worse as well.

If my story sounds familiar to you, I want you to know that those years were terrible for me. I was suffering greatly and I truly didn't know how I would ever recover. When you are in the darkness like I was, it seems like an impossible uphill battle to regain health and wellness. So if you are in a place right now like I was in, I see you, I understand you, I am you. And I am glad you are here because I am here to tell you that I was able to get myself out of that depression and ill health and today I feel amazing. I want to encourage you and let you know that if I can do it, you can do it too.

So there I was. Sick, depressed and unsure how I was going to be able to change my life. As I look back, I can honestly say that I knew what I had to do but I just wasn't doing it. Knowing what to do, therefore, was not the problem. I just didn't know how to do it.

I lived in a trying and failing vicious cycle. I was cycling between emotional states and engaging in self-destructive behaviors due to my emotional instability. I would go through periods where I tried to do something different but I always dropped out due to a lack of determination. The lack of strength, focus, motivation and conviction surfaced, so I ended up failing every time and this made me feel disappointed, guilty and hopeless. The more I failed, the more I lost the will to do anything at all. I was living every day of my life amid this whirlwind of negative emotions, watching the problems get worse and worse.

Oftentimes I would be lost in a whirlwind of negative thinking. At one of my worst moments, when I felt totally lost and desperate, I suddenly had the thought that I just wanted to be calm, to soothe the endless cycling thoughts in my head. It was at that moment that I finally realized and recognized that what I needed to do first and foremost was to calm my thoughts, calm my emotions and find my peace. In that moment, I was determined to find a way to do this and that is how I discovered meditation. I started meditating because I longed for just one moment of peace.

The amazing thing is that meditation did help me find that moment of peace and calm. Even more amazing is that to my surprise and immense joy, meditation also enabled me to find my strength.

So how did I do it? How did I add meditation into my life? Well, the truth is that I did not learn meditation overnight. It was a gradual process. Although I did feel the benefits from my first attempt at meditation, it took time for meditation to truly change my life. It was a slow, gradual change and with each new meditation my serenity grew and all the benefits of meditation began to manifest in my life.

As meditation became an everyday part of my life, my thoughts and feelings calmed down. Once that happened, I was able to begin to change the way I thought and eventually my thoughts became much more positive and uplifting. My thoughts actually supported me instead of harming me.

As my mind calmed down, I was able to connect with my deepest desires and to gain clarity and focus. I connected with the center of my being and felt peace. Once I did that, I discovered an inexhaustible source of inner strength that is with me always. I restructured my life and began to live in a way that made me feel good. I began to be the very best version of myself and everything that I did was aligned with my purpose.

Unexpectedly, when I was at my worst, I found meditation and through daily practice, I received all its benefits. Meditation helped me to conquer my health and now I teach meditation to others so they can use it on their own journeys. Based on my own personal experience and the results of others who have tried it, my recommendation for anyone on their own health journey is to learn meditation and make it part of your lifestyle.

Meditation is the first step on the journey of understanding yourself so that you can heal your body, mind and spirit.

HOW TO MEDITATE

Adding meditation into your life does not have to be complicated. Meditation is actually quite simple. It can be divided into four steps.

The first step is to learn a super basic, short form of meditation and start using it regularly at different times of the day. Beginning with a short meditation is the best way so that you can build the habit of meditation into your life until it becomes familiar.

The second step is to learn a natural passive form of meditation, in which you do not have to make any effort. This step allows you to continue to practice daily until you become comfortable in the meditative state.

At this point, you are already a meditator and you are receiving all the benefits of passive meditation, but the path can continue and from there, the third step is to increase the number and variety of practices to fully develop your ability and find your own meditation style.

Finally, the fourth step is to learn how to induce a quick meditative state at any time of the day and use it whenever you need it. I describe the suggested four steps of this learning process in more detail below so that you can easily put it into practice.

THE METHOD

Step 1: The Simplest Meditation: Sit up straight for a moment, close your eyes, take a deep breath and exhale slowly. Repeat this breath three to five times in a slow and relaxed way. Then open your eyes, smile and get on with your day.

Too simple? Exactly the point. It is simple and this is why it is the perfect starting point. This is a quick, simple meditation, but also very powerful. Give it a try and realize how different you feel after just five conscious breaths. Practice several times a day, for a few days until the feeling of meditation becomes familiar to you and then try step two.

Step 2. Natural Alpha State Passive Meditation: When you wake up first thing in the morning, sit up straight, close your eyes and breathe deeply and slowly for five minutes. Do not make any effort. Just allow the feeling of serenity and deep relaxation attributed to the natural alpha brain waves to take over while you continue to breathe calmly. Then open your eyes, smile and get on with your day.

What are alpha brain waves?

When you wake up your brain is producing alpha brain waves, which means you are awake, but not really focused on anything. You are naturally in a deep state of relaxation while in the alpha brain wave state. So, if you meditate first thing in the morning, you can take advantage of your natural brain condition upon awakening, which allows you to easily get into a deep meditative state. Then it will be easier to get used to the feeling of being present without thought, to sit calmly with a clear mind.

Wonderfully, when you meditate in an alpha state, you do not have to do anything but lie there relaxed, observing and enjoying each of your breaths from your awareness. You can start with five minutes each morning and gradually, as you feel more comfortable, increase the time.

Meditation first thing in the morning is a practice that you can maintain for the rest of your life. It will always bring you wonderful benefits. In my experience, it is the perfect way to start the day.

With practice, in addition to deep calm and relaxation, you will also experience interesting benefits related to intuition and creativity. By then, you will be able to use this deep meditative state to perform visualization exercises, which is known as active meditation and leads us to step three.

Step 3. Self-Induced Alpha State: Expand your meditation practice. Start meditating at other times and start trying other meditation techniques. Be curious and open to different types of meditation so you can discover your own meditation style.

Having mastered natural alpha meditation, it is time to develop your skill further and learn how to achieve a self-induced alpha state. Here opportunities expand greatly, but a good starting point would be to start meditating at other day times using the same process.

Just sit up straight, close your eyes and take a few deep breaths. You focus on reaching the desired meditative state. Stay relaxed and calm as you move into the meditative state. You are already used to it so you are training yourself to do it effortlessly. Meditating at other times of day will allow you to create calm spaces to recharge throughout the day and will bring an incredible sense of ease to your day.

When you have reached this point, you will be able to explore the meditation world more widely.

Consider that there are hundreds, if not thousands, of meditation techniques thanks to the great diversity of cultures and traditions around the world. My suggestion is to start doing guided meditations and visualizations which you can find online or on the multitude of meditation apps that are available. Gradually branch out and experiment with other meditation techniques, like deep breathing meditation, candle meditation, nature contemplation meditation, compassion meditation and forgiveness meditation. There are so many different meditations you can find online, so experiment until you find practices that really work for you. Make this a fun learning journey as you try different meditations.

Once you have found some meditations that work, you may want to take it a step further and learn advanced meditation techniques, such as Chakra Balancing Meditation, Tonglen Meditation, Microscopic Orbit Meditation, or the Silva Method Meditation. Remember to enjoy the process.

Regarding the advanced techniques, please note that advanced does not mean that they are more difficult, but that they require more instructions and steps and therefore you will have to study and learn them before you can use them.

In short, any type of meditation will help, because by this point you will have mastered the main thing, which is being able to reach a deep calm and relaxed state. So, my suggestion is to just keep curiously exploring and finding your own meditation style.

Step 4. Quick Meditative State: Learn to self-induce the meditative state in one breath. Simply breathe in and as you exhale connect with the deep sense of calm of the meditative state. Then smile and move on with your day. Practice during your daily activities throughout the day to bring awareness to the present moment.

At this point, you have so much practice that you can self-induce a deep meditative state quite quickly, whenever you want. Do this whenever you need to evoke a calm sensation. Anytime life is getting hectic or you notice your thoughts are beginning to spiral, remember to meditate. You can use the stressful feeling as a trigger to meditate. Do this by linking the idea that anytime you are feeling stressed out or your emotions are getting out of control, you can stop and meditate for one or two minutes to pull yourself out of the negativity.

Eventually you will train yourself to take a moment of peace anytime you need it.

Remember, meditation is a great practice in many situations. It can be used in a variety of circumstances where having a level head is necessary. Some examples of good times to meditate are: right before you have to make a decision, before you give an answer, directly prior to interacting with someone, when you have to give a speech or when your children or other family member is triggering you. You can take a moment of meditation in the middle of a meeting, during a discussion, or in any stressful situation. It will be just one second, but you will bring consciousness to your present moment in order to show up as your best self.

DOUBTS & LIMITING BELIEFS

Now, it may happen that, although the idea of meditating seems simple and reasonable to you, when considering the possibility of meditating you are assailed by doubts. This is very common. In fact, there are three very common doubts or limiting beliefs that people have when thinking about mediation. You may think meditation is not for you, you may have the belief that meditation is too hard or you may think that meditation takes too much time and you can't fit it into your schedule. Let's address each of them for you to help to clear some of these limiting beliefs.

The first limiting belief is thinking that meditation is not for you. For many reasons, you might not see yourself as a meditator. You may think that you are simply not the type to meditate or that meditation won't help you. The truth is that meditation is for absolutely everyone without exception, simply because meditation can bring benefits to all of us. If you are having this thought that meditation is not for you, I invite you to be curious and give it a try. Take it one day at a time with enthusiasm and discover what meditation can do for you. It may just change your life.

The second limiting belief is thinking that meditation is very difficult. Certainly, meditation has long been shrouded in a mystical atmosphere, but really, meditation is simply a skill that we all can learn and develop. In fact, you are already meditating throughout your day. Have you ever been driving and all of a sudden you look up and realize you don't even remember how you got to your destination? That's meditation. Or maybe you became engrossed in a hobby and time seemed to stand still. That's meditation. Or maybe you were looking at a rainbow or another amazing natural spot of beauty and you felt one with everything around you. That's meditation too.

You are already meditating unconsciously. Now you will be learning to meditate consciously and use it to bring a sense of peace into your life. I invite you to open to a new understanding of what meditation really is, realize that it can be a simple thing that does not need elaborate techniques or rituals and begin to practice and develop your skill progressively.

The third limiting belief is thinking that meditation takes a lot of time. This is partly true because as with every skill, practice makes perfect, but that does not mean that you must be an expert and master advanced meditation to receive its benefits.

In fact, it is just the opposite, you receive the benefits of meditation even if you only meditate for a short time. As you continue to meditate, you will see that you are able to achieve deeper and deeper benefits as your mind becomes calmer and calmer. Give yourself a chance to add meditation to your life and focus on practicing consistently. It can be just five deep breaths at any time of the day, or five minutes every morning, but if you practice consistently, you will soon see results and love them.

PRACTICE

Now if you are ready to start, we are going to practice step one together.

We are going to do the Simplest Meditation right now. Take your time, there is no rush. There is also no desired result, just experience it. Remember, just sit up straight for a moment, close your eyes, take a deep breath and exhale slowly. Repeat the breath three to five times in a slow and relaxed way. Then open your eyes, smile and continue reading. Do it now.

Congratulations! You have just meditated!

How was it? Do you notice any changes? Remember, this is only your first brief meditation. You will notice greater benefits as you continue meditating. For now, celebrate that you started. The first step is always the hardest.

Now, set a date to begin practicing step two, the Natural Alpha State Passive Meditation. Set your alarm five minutes earlier than your usual time. When your alarm goes off, sit up straight, close your eyes and breathe deeply and slowly for five minutes.

Keep practicing consistently, keep experiencing meditation at whatever level you are at each day, without expectations. Just allow yourself to enjoy the experience. Take note of any positive results you see. Does your mind calm down? Is the feeling of overwhelm disappearing? Does your stress level seem to have gone down? Notice the changes and use them as motivation to continue to build your meditation practice.

As you continue to meditate, you may find that you are able to remain focused and aligned with your true goals and desires. Gradually, the doubts will fall away and you will be aware of your strength. You will be able to overcome anything as you calm your mind and build your confidence in your own ability to control yourself.

This is the first step on your healing journey. Once you master your mind, you can overcome anything, including any challenge in your journey of conquering health.

Mediation has helped me immensely and it can help you too if you are willing to give it a chance. Meditation will not cure you, but it will transform you into a person capable of doing what is necessary to overcome all your health problems.

I hope that by making meditation part of your lifestyle, you transform yourself from someone who is overwhelmed, frustrated and self-doubting, into someone serene and centered, with self-control and inner strength to overcome all challenges throughout your health transformation journey.

As you embrace the path of meditation, I wish you success on your journey. If you have been inspired to start meditating and wish to connect, I would absolutely love to hear from you. After all, we are all walking this path together.

Quiet the mind and the soul will speak.
~ **MA JAYA SATI BHAGAVATI**

ABOUT THE AUTHOR

Claudia Valentinuzzi Núñezi is a food engineer with a long professional career in diverse fields such as research, quality, innovation, entrepreneurship and business development. Her passions are learning and helping. Life forced her to learn about health-related topics, to help herself and her loved ones, but then also allowed her to become a certified health and fitness coach which was a turning point in her life.

Through coaching she has been able to combine her strengths and help people who really need it, in a practical, effective and above all loving way. Claudia's signature is passion and dedication. She has always been committed to excellence in everything she does, and coaching is no exception. As a coach, she focuses on inspiring others to take good care of themselves and enrich their lives with love and kindness.

Contact Information:
Linkedin: https://www.linkedin.com/in/claudiavalentinuzzi/

If you were all alone in the universe
with no one to talk to,
no one with which to share the beauty of the stars,
to laugh with, to touch, what would
be your purpose in life?
It is other life, it is love, which
gives your life meaning.
This is harmony.
We must discover the joy of each other,
the joy of challenge, the joy of growth."

~Mitsugi Saotome

CHAPTER 22

EVERYDAY GRATITUDE & THE BALANCE OF STRUCTURE AND FLEXIBILITY

by Nancy Yang Timmins

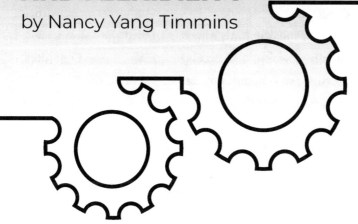

TOPIC:	MIndset
TOOL:	Gratitude
TECHNIQUE:	Each day, reflect on the things you are grateful for. As you go through your day, notice all the things you have to be grateful for and begin to feel that gratitude towards all aspects of life.

No duty is more urgent than giving thanks.

~ J O H N A L L E N

It has only been a year and a half since I embarked on this journey of transforming my health, but I cannot even remember where I was on the health continuum before now. I feel at home with how I am living my life now. It feels like it has always been this way, flowing with ease. I had to return to my first gratitude journal entry to jog my memory.

Where was I before? Well, let's begin before the pandemic, more than two and a half years ago.

I was burned out and stressed out. As a stay-at-home mom with a husband who traveled frequently for business, I carried the entire weight of my family's well-being, health and success on my shoulders. I felt like I was expected to do this, even though no one had ever told me I had to. I was there for everyone in my family and I didn't really take care of myself.

I took care of my family, but I also volunteered at my kids' schools and helped out at their various sports events. I enjoyed helping others because it felt good and it also gave me a chance to get out of the house and meet other adults. But more selfishly, I got to see and know what was happening at their schools and sports.

I was on the road a lot, driving my kids to their schools, their sports practices, their competitions and other extracurricular activities. When I wasn't doing that, I was going to my volunteering commitments and organizing everyone's schedule so I could fit everything in.

I also had to run a household with all that entails. Cooking, cleaning, organizing, doing laundry. It was a lot of work. Besides the responsibilities at home, my responsibilities at my volunteer positions were always increasing. I got more and more involved and I was extremely busy. Being busy was like a status symbol to me, a way for me to prove my value.

The downside to all of this was that I wasn't taking care of myself. I always put others ahead of myself and I ended up neglecting my own needs and well-being.

I have scoliosis and have had chronic back pain for years. I knew it was important to take care of my physical body, but I never paid much attention to it. Others' needs always came before my own.

I did see various professionals for my back issue. I saw chiropractors, a physiotherapist, a massage therapist and even an acupuncturist on a regular basis. This was a normal part of my life. I outsourced the help I needed but never once thought I had the power to change my situation. I had the My-Body-Is-Not-My-Business mindset. It was the "I'm paying these health-care professionals so much money that they should help me" and "this is the best I can do" thinking.

There are limitations in what a health-care professional can do for us because they are specialized in their respective field and they treat only one aspect of the body. They concentrate on the problem presented without looking at the whole body as one.

A far better approach is to examine the body as a whole. To take a holistic approach to health: physical, emotional, mental and spiritual. Our body has different needs. There is no one-size-fits-all pill or prescription. Additionally, each person is different, each body is different, so each person has different needs. It is essential to determine for ourselves what works best for us. We must take responsibility for our health.

I did not take responsibility for my health and this made me a victim of my own negative thoughts, patterns and behaviors.

There were things I did for my health, but it was always within various constraints I placed upon myself. I did walk a lot, as it was the cheapest and easiest exercise option for I did not want to spend 'my husband's' money. I also did yoga for years because I heard it would help people with their back pain. I enjoyed both yoga and walking, however, these exercises did not decrease my reliance on my health-care team.

I also tried countless 'fitness crazes' like Barre Yoga, Hot Yoga, Pilates and Kick Boxing with the goal of building more cardio-strength and looking more 'toned'. They helped somewhat, but not enough. I didn't feel toned or fit. My back pain would still throw me off the flow frequently. Something was missing.

Finally, in my early 40's I realized that resistance training was important, especially for women. I knew it was an essential element in avoiding illnesses like osteoporosis and sarcopenia. My mom had been diagnosed with osteoporosis, so I was well aware of the dangers of not taking care of my fitness. I made the decision to do something to ensure I wouldn't end up with a similar diagnosis when I got older. At the age of 42, I started to work out with a trainer at the gym. I worked with her for about nine months and then I created a workout program for myself that I continued with.

My workout program became quite demanding. I went from working out two or three days a week to five or six days a week. I was spending an hour and a half to two hours each session at the gym. My time at the gym was taking away the quality time that I could spend with my family or completing my daily tasks and fulfilling my responsibilities. I was feeling guilty. I was also not seeing the results with the amount of time I was putting in. I was exhausted, tired, resentful and I felt under-appreciated for all that I did. Then the pandemic hit.

I was happy for the down time. Although it was a stressful time in many ways, for me, being 'trapped' at home meant that I did not have to drive around like a chicken with its head cut off and I finally had some time for myself.

My kids were 11 and 15 at this point so they didn't need me all the time. They were in virtual schools and could handle their own schoolwork and their own schedules. I was still involved on the Board level at my son's swim club and the board meetings continued during the pandemic, but it was a lot less time volunteering than I normally did.

My son was swimming on and off whenever the lockdown was lifted and my daughter was paddling in the summertime when it was all out-doors, however, this was a lot less of a commitment than before. The endless driving to activities had lessened and was much more manageable during the pandemic since most things were closed. I got more down time than pre-pandemic, because of online schooling and online training sessions for kids during lockdowns.

I started it off like everyone else. I binged watched. I indulged in my fantasy novel reading. I went to bed late. There was some structure in my life, but it was based on my kids' schedules and my volunteer schedules. I continued to work out at the gym and at home during lockdowns.

And then, things began to change. My husband and I started going for walks every day, rain or shine or snow, just for a chance to get out of the house. We did this for almost the entire first year of the pandemic. We would chat and discuss where we saw our family going, our kids going, where his career was going and what I would do after the kids grew up and moved out of the house. We bought more self-help books, which we have not finished reading. The turning point, for my rapid health transformation, came when we discovered personal growth. We began down the path of learning and it has been life changing.

I began to learn about habits and routines. I realized I needed to give my life more structure, so I created a schedule for myself that incorporated a lot of the techniques I was learning. One of the best things I learned about was to practice gratitude.

GRATITUDE PRACTICE

On January 17, 2021 I decided to start writing in a gratitude journal. Little did I know then that this would be a practice that would change my mindset and ultimately, change my life.

Starting something new is always hard and that was the case for my gratitude journal. I did not know what to write. My aim for perfection got in the way. I wanted to write things that really touched my heart and I felt deeply about. I could only write about one thing initially. That was our health, as my family and the fact that we were all healthy during the pandemic. After about six days and casting perfectionism aside, it seemed that my attention was redirected and grateful thoughts started to flood in. I was easily able to write in my gratitude journal each day.

I went through a very intense period of learning. I dove into a variety of personal growth topics which was amazing and even better, taking these courses gave me the opportunity to meet lots of other like-minded individuals.

Here's the amazing thing: the more I discovered about myself, the more grateful I was towards everything in my life. There was no lack of material for my gratitude journal. It slowed me down further and helped me to become more aware of what had always been working perfectly for us. Many things that worked before the pandemic continued to work. The world did not stop because we were 'trapped' inside our homes. Grocery stores continued to run. Pharmacies continued to open. School was still happening, even though it was now online. People were still working, although from home. Hospitals and front-line workers continued to put their lives at risk for us. I was able to stop focusing on What-I-Did-Not-Have and I began focusing on What-Was-Already-Given-To-Me.

EXPANDING YOUR GRATITUDE JOURNAL

I kept writing in my gratitude journal and it evolved over time. Soon my gratitude journal became an 'emotions' journal, too. For the first time I was tuning into what I was grateful for and this allowed me to tap into my emotions in a different way than ever before. I learned so much about myself from this practice.

Once I began to write down my emotions, I was able to reflect on why certain circumstances triggered a strong reaction within me. Even when a negative emotion arose, I was able to write something positive about why I was grateful for it. I began to understand that negative emotions were not really negative, they were simply information about how we feel.

An example of this happened with my daughter and I. We had gotten into an argument over why she didn't want to continue paddling. I felt she should continue because she excelled in it. As the argument continued, I observed myself getting frustrated. Instead of reacting right away, I used some of the new tools I had learned and instead, I took a few deep breaths before walking away. I was proud of myself because the old me would have reacted right away, but I did not this time. That was a win.

Walking away gave both of us time to think about what had happened. When the topic came up again, my daughter expressed her dislikes for competitive sports. I, with my ego speaking as a mom who wanted to show off her kids' accomplishments, just could not understand her reasoning. "Why?" I said, "You are so good at it." "I just don't like it or enjoy it," she replied firmly.

After everyone went to bed and I was alone with my gratitude journal, I began to write about my emotions. I was still a bit frustrated but this was my gratitude journal so I directed my attention to the positive, "I'm grateful for my daughter being true to herself and expressing her true feelings with me. I'm grateful that she is not a pushover. As her guide to her experience on Earth, I need to respect her wishes."

Wow! I was shocked when I looked down to see what I had written. That was a huge awakening for me when I finally realized how there is a silver lining to everything. We never raised the topic about her doing competitive sports again in our house which meant there were no more arguments on the topic. It was so simple, but this approach would never have occurred to me before I had discovered personal growth.

Keeping the gratitude journal has enabled me to be more present, since my attention stays focused on the things I am grateful for each day. This totally changed me. I was feeling less resentful, calmer and happier. I noticed that I was starting to be a lot less angry and have less emotional outbreaks. I was sleeping better, feeling less stressed and was getting better results with my workout program.

My relationships with my family were better all around. Before I started gratitude journal keeping, I was the person who would be calm most of the time and would blow up suddenly. I would feel so terrible and guilty after the emotional eruption that I needed to apologize to my family. The emotional outbursts are happening a lot less frequently now. I still have some challenges and may get a little more tense with my word choices, but I'm better at riding the emotional wave, observing it and letting it recede. I am getting better at not reacting. I have learned to take a breath to give myself time to respond appropriately to each situation that comes up.

SCHEDULING

*Schedule it, whatever it is that we
want to do or spend time on*

~ JIM KWIK

I saw this quote and it rang true for me. I decided to take this advice. I decided to use Google Calendar to plan my days. It has helped me to be more organized and to plan the things I want to do instead of just racing through my days trying to accomplish what I need to in a random way. I am so grateful for the creativity of the human mind that came up with the abundance of technology and tools which make our lives easier. Google Calendar is one.

I had used a calendar in the past, but I had only used it for my kids' activity schedules and appointments and my husband's schedule. I had nothing for myself at all. Basically, I did not plan my days except for the plans of my kids and husband. As I took stock of what regular things, tasks and errands I would like to do and that I needed to do, I thought deeply about how I wanted to spend my days. I wanted to incorporate the new health practices and exercise protocols I had learned into my daily and weekly life so I organized them all with Google Calendar, without feeling guilty that I was blocking those times out. I was finally putting myself on the list. I was much more organized too, because I set reminders for myself so I wouldn't forget my appointments.

This system gave me an overview of my day and the week ahead. I made sure that I added breaks in between the activities and tasks so I wouldn't feel like I was busy all the time. Putting everything into a calendar relieved me of unnecessary stress and worries. It also allowed flexibility in my schedule because life can be unpredictable. On my calendar I made sure that the things that I must get done like daily meditation were on the schedule and I also gave myself flexibility around less important things, I gave myself the flexibility to shift things as the day unfolded. I became less rigid, allowing myself to understand that I did not have to complete everything on my to-do list if the day didn't end up as planned.

Scheduling some time for myself to rest and recover was essential. This was so much easier now because my days and weeks were organized. I did not need to make sacrifices or treat myself like a martyr anymore. I did not need to validate my self-worth with my sacrifice or contribution. I recognized that when we did so much for others, we would deprive them of learning how to take care of themselves. This is an essential skill.

PRIORITIZING HEALTH

Health is our first wealth. Our bodies have been there with us since birth, or even before birth and our bodies continue to be with us until the last moment of our lives. Our body is truly a miraculous masterpiece. I have learned to appreciate this beautiful vessel that is here to allow me to fully experience the ups and downs of my human life. I love how my body allows me to love, to grow, to experiment, to play and to feel through my senses and my emotions. I am grateful for my body. I wish I had appreciated my body long ago. The truth is, we should all be grateful for our bodies, no matter where we are on the journey. Loving our bodies today can help us take care of it in a way that will nourish us and allow us to live our best lives for all the days of our life.

FINAL WORDS

Keeping a gratitude journal has opened my eyes to the beauty and abundance around me. It has opened my heart to receive and to share. Keeping a gratitude journal has re-established my connection to others, to my body, to my spirit and to the universe.

I have come to believe that we are all students here on earth. We are in the school of life together. Keeping my gratitude journal has allowed me to strengthen my connections to all of my fellow students in the "How to

Be a Better Human" school of planet Earth. This might seem like a silly way to approach it, but if you allow yourself to let the sentiment sink in, you might just change the way you approach life.

It is possible to take charge of your health and to create a better life for yourself. It all starts with gratitude. Being grateful for where you are today is the key to it all.

I leave you with this: Today, I am an entirely new person. I am healthier, happier, calmer and more loving than I was before I started on this journey. My first step was taken with starting a gratitude journal.

Are you ready to give it a try? What have you got to lose?

With gratitude,
Nan

I would maintain that thanks are the highest form of thought; and that gratitude is happiness doubled by wonder

~ G.K. CHESTERTON

ABOUT THE AUTHOR

Nan was a stay-at-home mom of two for 17 years before she became a certified health coach. She holds certifications in HoloBody & 10X Fitness Coach. Her transformational journey included working through a variety of personal growth courses on the Mindvalley platform. She was inspired by these courses, which prompted her to take the health certifications. She was amongst the first trained Holobody coaches and was one of the first 20 people to graduate from the 10X Coaching Certification Program.

Nan is in the best shape of her life now at 47, all thanks to the tools and practices that she has been able to learn and incorporate into her life. For someone who could not be found online prior to completing her certifications, she now has a blog, a website, a public Instagram account, a Facebook account and a LinkedIn account.

She continues to be active in the HoloBody and 10X Coaching Community and frequently shares her insights from her coaching practice with fellow coaches. The key to her success is her authenticity and genuine care and love towards others.

She believes that collaboration and co-elevation is the key to raising the collective consciousness in this next evolutionary chapter of Human History.

Contact Information:
Blog: followthejaderabbit.com
Instagram: @timyanan
LinkedIn: www.linkedin.com/in/nancy-yang-timmins-holistichealthandfitness
YouTube: Health Simplified with Nan

Just like an electric plant generates electricity, you can generate happiness from within.

~Irina Shehovsov

CHAPTER 23
TEN MINUTES OF JOY

by Irina Shehovsov

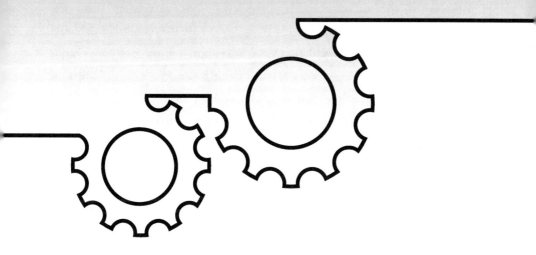

TOPIC:	Mindfulness
TOOL:	Ten Minutes of Joy
TECHNIQUE:	Whenever you are feeling overwhelmed, take ten minutes to do something that brings you joy.

To be joyful is a principle. It doesn't change with emotions. Joy is an inner contentment despite all the circumstances.

~ RICHARD DALY

Total health is when you experience health in all states of being. It is when your physical, emotional, mental and spiritual states are all in alignment. All systems must thrive in order to create the extraordinary experience of living the healthiest life you can while here on planet Earth.

My health journey began when my world fell apart. It is interesting that it took an event where one part of my life was ending before I woke up to the realization that I had to change everything. Why is it that we often wait until the worst happens before we recognize we must do something? It is most likely that we become complacent. We think, "Well, if it isn't broken, don't fix it." Even if we aren't fully happy or healthy, we often don't realize we need to do something different. When an event occurs that throws you down onto your knees, it can push you into taking action.

The event that started my health journey was a breakup. It was unexpected. Suddenly, I found myself becoming a single parent of two. It was a terrible time for me. I was living in misery and waiting for someone to come rescue me. I was barely holding on. I felt like I was bringing my best self to work and my kids would get the leftovers. Although I was doing the best I could, I felt that my children deserved more and that I deserved more.

I realized that my current state of living no longer worked. I didn't buy into the idea that we come here to suffer and I wanted to discover something better for my family. This was the moment where I decided to take action. This was when I started my journey to recover the pieces of my broken self so I could become happy and healthy again. Since there was no-one to help me and nobody to care of me now, it was my job to do so myself. What I discovered along the way has truly been eye opening.

Some things are simple, yet we take them for granted. As I began my journey, I found a system of living where I could combine my physical, emotional, mental and spiritual health. The system was one where I viewed myself as a whole person. I knew I needed to take care of all aspects of myself and along the way, I learned how important it is to create healthy habits.

You are what you repeatedly do. You must be consistent as you seek improvement. Creating healthy habits for living allows you to experience the best life possible. You have this one body and this one lifetime so it is essential that you take good care of it. Your body provides so much abundance. It breathes, it makes the heart beat, it walks, it jumps, it swims, it runs. All of these activities use energy so it is important to exercise, eat right and protect your body from harm.

My journey started with a simple walk outside. For some reason, on that day, I felt like a baby who is just learning to walk, full of curiosity about the world around them. Amazed at what is possible. It was like I was seeing with new eyes that were able to take in the wonder all around me.

After that first walk there was no going back. That walk was the ignition that I needed to get me going. The walk made me want to add more activities into my life that sparked this joy of living. And thus, I began to add activities and little by little, I created a morning routine which was and is incredible. I now love my mornings; I no longer feel dread about waking up each day. It is truly an awesome time of day to set the intention, to practice gratitude and forgiveness, to meditate, to learn something new and to sing my heart out.

Of course, I did not stumble upon it by accident, I was adding each component, one at a time. I was learning more about myself and the world and as part of that, I was determined to discover the best tools I could find that would help me feel alive, energized, uplifted and motivated. As I learned the tools, I added them into my daily routine. It is one thing to learn something and it is another when you make it a part of your life. When you add it to your life and practice it, you make it your own.

Some things were easy, others were challenging. But I kept on. During the process, I had moments where I doubted myself, where I wondered if I was making any progress, but I soldiered on. Forward, forward, ever forward. After a few months, I looked at my life and realized I had changed completely, my life had changed completely. I felt like a new person. Looking back, I can connect the dots and see how much had changed. Things that used to bother me no longer did. I was calm and relaxed most of the time. I was no longer feeling like a victim. I had taken control of my life.

There are many tools I learned along the way, but I would like to dedicate this chapter to a tool that is fun, easy to do and which helps you keep joy and fun at the center of your life.

Happiness is at the core of our health. When we are happier, we become healthier. One radical idea about total health that I want to introduce is the idea of buidling a happiness muscle. We all know we need to exercise, eat right, get enough sleep and reduce our stress, but what we often forget is that we also need to experience happiness in order to have a truly spectacular life.

Total health would not be complete if we leave out our emotional health. The idea of a happiness muscle is a tool you can have in your pocket, like a building block, to use as a pick me up that brightens your day. Like everything in life, if you want to improve something, you must practice it, you must make it a habit. We all have habits like brushing our teeth and taking a shower, eating and drinking. What if we create a habit of experiencing and maintaining joy and happiness in our life?

We do not need to wait to be happy when a milestone is crossed. We don't have to wait until a deal is done, or the promotion comes through or the person you wanted also wants you. We can choose to be happy now.

Think about what would happen if you could be happy now. Because you can be. You can choose to be happy right now, this second.

The truth is that each one of us gets to decide how we want to feel. We decide if we are going to feel happy or sad, excited or calm, bright or gloomy. We each get to choose our own experience of life. We always have a choice how we react to something. We choose.

This might seem like an extreme idea. After all, what about when things go wrong, when life gets rough? We all know that life is not unicorns and rainbows all the time. Tough events do happen, but in those moments, we make a choice about how we want to respond to these events. The choices that we make will influence our decisions and shape our lives. Our choices help to create our beliefs about the world and what we consider to be true. Why not choose how we respond so that we can deal with all events in our lives, even difficult ones, with ease and grace?

The truth is that we often seek external happiness. We say we will get happy when some event or another occurs, when some person or another approves of us, when we hit some successful moment we can revel in. And yes, those moments do bring happiness, but did you ever notice that it only lasts for a short time? Before long we are looking forward once again, waiting for the next big thing to make us happy.

It's time to change our mindset. To remember one simple fact. The fact that true happiness lies within. Just like an electric plant generates electricity, we can generate our own happiness. Notice the word generate. Generate means it is created by us, not from some external source. We have all the resources and tools necessary to produce it. Our amazing body and its equally amazing natural chemical factory can create happiness on demand. When you generate happiness from within, it lasts. We have an inexhaustible supply of this happiness inside of each of us, just waiting to be discovered.

TEN MINUTES OF JOY

I would like to promote the habit of happiness as one of the keys to good health. One of the easiest ways to get started is to practice ten minutes of joy each day. It is simple, it is easy, it is sustainable. All you have to do is spend ten minutes each day doing something that sets your soul on fire! Imagine that you can change your emotional state in just ten minutes! And when you change your emotional state, it positively impacts your health. When you are happy, all parts of your life improve.

When I began to practice my ten minutes of joy, I discovered joy in singing. It was the best possible thing I could have done for myself and it really helped me to recover from the breakup. Singing allowed me to sing what I could not speak. I was not great at it in the beginning, but I kept on singing. Like any skill, I practiced and became better and better. I noticed the changes in my ability and that made me want to do it even more. Using this tool added zest and vigor to my life. When I practice singing for ten minutes or more, I feel joy, happiness and elation. I become completely involved, present in the moment and the time seems to fly by.

When you cultivate a habit that you enjoy, you are sending a signal to your brain that what you are doing is important. When you enjoy something, the chemical factory in your brain starts producing amazing hormones like endorphins, oxytocin, dopamine and serotonin. These are hormones that make you feel good which makes you want to repeat it again and again. This is how you create a habit.

FINDING YOUR TEN MINUTES OF JOY

If it has been a while or you are not sure what your passion or joy is, it is never too late to find out.

Is there something you wanted to try or learn for the longest time but never found the time? Why not start now? Or perhaps you used to do a hobby but you stopped? Now is a good time to revisit that hobby. It might still be enjoyable for you. Or is there a sport you are interested in doing? Add that into your life. Even a short ten minute trial can be fun.

Explore different avenues until you find something you enjoy. Add spark back into your life. It is all up to you. What would make you happy? Take charge and remember that happiness is at the core of your health.

ACTION STEPS

Here are some action steps to bring *Ten Minutes of Joy* into your life:

- Block out the same time on your calendar for ten minutes or more each day. Take your schedule into consideration and make sure it is a time when you can consistently practice.
- Do the activity. Pick something that involves a skill or is a challenge.
- There are many different activities to choose from, pick one from this list or create your own:
  - Singing
  - Playing a musical instrument
  - Writing
  - Baking/Cooking
  - Painting
  - Dancing
  - Learning a Foreign Language
  - Do a crossword puzzle
  - Do a jigsaw puzzle
  - Spending a few minutes with a loved one
- As you begin to practice your *Ten Minutes of Joy*, go easy on yourself. Don't give up if you are struggling in the beginning. Keep at it. Continue practicing every day for a few weeks to let the habit set in.
- When you are trying something new, give it at least seven days before you decide to switch to a different activity. It sometimes takes time to get used to doing something new. We often feel better about something once our skill improves.
- Enjoy the process as you master the skill.
- Remember to practice everyday to fill your days with joy.

I usually practice this habit in the afternoons. This serves as a reset point, especially because I work all day and I like to have a break before my children need my attention.

After my breakup, I was on a quest to find happiness. I wanted to be content again. I was searching on the outside, but I couldn't find true happiness until I came to understand that it was an inside job. Since I have been practicing happiness, I am in better health than I have been since I was a young woman. Every area of life has improved tremendously. Having a happiness practice gives me the energy I need to create other healthy habits.

HEALTHY HABITS: PHYSICAL HEALTH

For physical health, it is nutrition, movement and rest.

Avoid diets or quick fix routines. Instead, focus on changing your identity and making lifestyle changes. When you do something because this is who you are and this is the life you want to live, it is much easier to sustain positive changes.

Nutrition means having a sustainable whole food diet consisting of fruits, vegetables and proteins. This will reduce cravings. Use food as fuel, nothing more nothing less. Think of the food you eat in terms of whether it is going to support the body you desire.

Our bodies were designed to move. Whether this is a formal exercise routine in a gym or active sports and hobbies, get moving! You get to choose what movement. Once I started to add movement into my life, I decided to get a health coaching certification to learn even more. I am now a certified health coach and I delight in helping others on their journey. In addition to teaching my clients how to eat and exercise properly for their body type, I teach them to add *Ten Minutes of Joy* into their lives. My clients have consistently reported that building their happiness muscle helps them create healthy habits in all areas of their life.

There are other physical practices that will be helpful. Simple practices include getting enough sleep and going to bed at the same time each day; refraining from eating three hours prior to sleep and turning off all technology at least two hours before sleep.

For mental and emotional health, it is meditation, forgiveness, gratitude practice and of course, *Ten Minutes of Joy*.

It is the habits we create and which we sustain daily that allow us to have inner peace and happiness. This is subtle, it cannot be seen or heard, but only felt. Having these practices reduces stress and anxiety, eliminates anger and frustration and builds up your inner resilience to address life challenges.

Meditation creates clarity, peace and ease throughout your day. There are countless meditation techniques you could learn, so try out a few and find one that works for you. You can also download a meditation app on your phone and you will find that these apps have meditations that can fit into any lifestyle. From meditations that last five minutes to over an hour, you will find a meditation that works for you.

Forgiveness allows you to live without baggage. Every day when you interact with people, notice when you feel upset. If someone or something happens that throws you off and makes you angry, take notice. Then, actively practice forgiving that person or event. Do not carry this into another day. Forgive today to create a better tomorrow. Remember, forgiveness is a gift you give yourself.

Gratitude shows that no matter how difficult or unfortunate a situation is, there are always things to be grateful for. It could be small things, like being able to walk, breathe, have food on the table and a roof over your head. Learn to notice all the things you have to be grateful for. Even waking up each day is something to be grateful for. Practicing gratitude helps you to concentrate on the things that are working in your life and the more you focus on this, the better your life becomes.

Ten Minutes of Joy is the crown jewel and highlight of any day, an added benefit, especially if you feel sad, stagnant or drudging through the day. Do not delay. Add this amazing practice into your day today and start building your happiness muscle!

The above habits do not happen overnight. Take one at a time and build each habit into your life. Make it a deliberate and conscious creation. One thing at a time, one micro movement in the direction of the goal.

FINAL WORDS

When I began this journey, my goal was to take full responsibility for myself and my life. I wanted to create a better life for myself and my children. I set out to create a life where I am energetic, alive, healthy, vibrant and ready to create in other areas of my life.

What I have learned is that I have this one body and one lifetime. It is up to me to make sure that I take good care of the vehicle that allows me to have the greatest human experience possible.

My life changed in incredible ways because I improved my health. It all started with that walk where I experienced my ten minutes of joy.

Today, I am excited to wake up each morning to welcome a new day, to practice my morning routine, not because I have to but because I want to. When I shifted my mindset, I changed my life. It wasn't about a quick fix, but rather about changing who I am.

My wish for you is that you take a journey towards health and wellness. Whether you want to lose weight, quit smoking, save money or improve your relationships, taking the time to practice your own *Ten Minutes of Joy* will help you get where you are going.

Remember, you are changing who you are. Once you do that, you will easily be able to create habits and make choices in line with your new persona. The person you are being would determine the actions, thoughts and emotions that go with that. If you were an Olympic athlete, would you snack on junk food? If you were a writer, would you only write once in a while? No, you would do what you needed to do to excel in your area of expertise. Once you change who you are, you will be able to make the right choices too.

You know what is good for you. You know what you want. I am here to tell you that you can get there. If I was able to, anyone is able to. All it takes is the decision that you want to change, that you want a better life for yourself.

Do yourself a favor and practice *Ten Minutes of Joy* and see your life improve! It would give me immense joy to hear from you. Please reach out to me to share your successes with your practice of *Ten Minutes of Joy*.

With Love and Joy,
Irina

> *Think joy, talk joy, practice joy, share joy, saturate your mind with joy and you will have the time of your life today and every day all your life.*
> **~NORMAN VINCENT PEALE**

⚙️ ABOUT THE AUTHOR

Irina Shehovsov is the Founder of Reclaim Your Life and a #1 International Best Selling Author. She believes just like an electric plant generates electricity, you can generate happiness from within, which is a daily practice. Irina is Certified NLP Trainer, Time Line Therapy™ and Hypnotherapy Master Coach, Certified Wellness Coach and a 10X Fitness Coach.

By taking a holistic 360-degree approach, she focuses on restoring her clients physical, emotional, mental and spiritual states of being. Happiness Academy is her mentorship program that helps women remember who they are after a toxic relationship. Irina supports single parents in becoming better versions of themselves by sharing powerful stories on her podcast, *Single Parent Success Stories.*

She also coaches entrepreneurs on how to use the power of their mind to produce exponential growth in their business and profitability.

Irina's intention is to empower women to believe in themselves, no matter what anyone says.

Irina lives in Long Island NY with her two wonderful children. She has created a joyous life for her family using the tools she learned along the way.

Contact Information:
Email: irina@irinashehovsov.com
Website: https://www.irinashehovsov.com
Instagram: https://www.instagram.com/re.claimyourlife/

I am the wisest man alive, for I know one thing, and that is that I know nothing.

~Plato, The Republic

No one is free who has not obtained the empire of himself.

~Pythagoras

CHAPTER 24

SELF INQUIRY A LOGIC SKILL FOR FREEDOM

by André Roggy

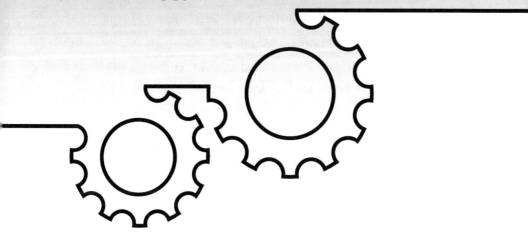

TOPIC:	Self Knowledge
TOOL:	Self Inquiry
TECHNIQUE:	When you have a disempowering thought or belief, challenge yourself by asking yourself a series of questions to determine if what you believe is actually true.

What lies behind us and what lies before us are tiny matters compared to what lies within us.

~ RALPH WALDO EMERSON

I grew up in the Midwest United States. I was the youngest child of three and from my earliest memories, I simply didn't feel like I fit in. I am the one who didn't look like any of my siblings or the people around me and I stood out, not only amongst my family, but around seemingly everyone. I didn't fully comprehend why or in what ways I was different, I just knew.

As I got older, I began to observe the ways that I was different from others. The more obvious were the jet-black hair and pale skin amongst all the blond-haired and tanned neighbors. I was much shorter than the people in my neighborhood as well and my shorter stature made me feel insecure. The less obvious were my intense shyness coupled with old-soul precociousness. It was an odd combination for a child and one that made me stand out even more.

My parents, having had their try at two children before me, did their best to efficiently educate me for worldly success. I trusted their guidance and obeyed their rules since I was finding it difficult to navigate the world with my otherness. I wanted to be told how to act and how to be so that I could finally fit in.

One afternoon in my early youth, I blindly trusted my older sister when she told me to touch a hot curling iron. Burned for my naïveté, both figuratively and literally, you would think I would have grown up into an anti-establishmentarian, questioning rebel. At the time, however, it just made me distrust my siblings and peers, which made me trust my parents' guidance even more.

I was eager to please my emotionally unavailable father so I obeyed him blindly. I feared not following his stern warnings about how I should act. My father believed that I was generally "overly sensitive" and I would often hear him worriedly telling my mother that I was a "cry baby" and "momma's boy." This made me feel terrible and made me cower as I feared expressing my feelings. I ended up suppressing them, stuffing down the otherness I had felt my entire life. I didn't want to be a cry baby or a momma's boy so I did my best to be what my father wanted instead.

I never had a chance to truly understand my feelings at all. I tried to ignore them, to pretend I didn't feel the way I did. I didn't learn to deal with my emotions effectively at all. I knew that in order to survive, I had to "man up," which meant that my emotions had to be stuffed down, the otherness, the undesirable feelings. I had to become someone else.

This was when I learned that I had to follow the rules if I was going to be 'normal'. I learned how to blindly trust rules and teachings. They were safe. They were my keys to survival. I learned to conform, perform and people please. I learned to turn my back on who I really was so I could fit into the group.

It wasn't until I'd gone twenty odd years of repression, subservience and fitting in that I finally met a truly wise teacher. She was my opera and classical singing coach but she became a lot more than that to me. She became almost like a second mother and helped me learn the art of living and being courageous by embracing my true, authentic self.

I will be honest with you, there were times that I thought I had met a real life witch, since she had crystal ball clarity to see things about me and within me I thought no-one could have known these things about me otherwise.

It was with my opera coach's encouragement that I finally saw a therapist who diagnosed me as chronically depressed. Hearing the D word slowly shocked me into the realization that I had been vacillating between numbness, anxiety and suicidal ideation most of my life. I had been so out of touch with how I really felt that I hadn't even realized how deep my pain went. Although there had been times of hope, happiness and love, they were always closely accompanied by fear, limiting beliefs, perfectionism, expectation and conditionality.

My teacher gave me the courage to embrace my traits of otherness and learn what was right for me. Her therapeutic skills of mirroring and gentle insight helped me start the process of breaking down my facade that I had been rotting within. The licensed therapist helped me start to unravel the tangled web of emotion, thought and history inside that edifice. Working with both of them, I started to wake up to the lies I'd been telling myself and others that kept me on such a limited, inauthentic and destructive path.

That is when my life began to turn around. When I began to question my beliefs about myself, others and situations, I was able to see that I had lived with a limiting mindset. I set out to learn tools to help me understand what was true and what was not true. This process has been the most powerful transformational tool I have found for leaving behind a life that doesn't work for you and stepping into the life you were meant to live.

BELIEF & PERCEPTION

Modern humans generally learn to run in life before they can even walk. The brain, psyche and our emotions are powerful tools and we are just beginning to comprehend how they work. So few of us learn to master them, even after a lifetime.

Youth has the grand opportunity to develop the skills of perception, to understand one's place and connection to the world and to learn to command and grasp not only the body, but also the mind and emotions. However, the young are generally influenced by the adults around them as well as the expectations, rituals and beliefs of their society. Cultural values are more subtle, but also weave in and out of such indoctrinations.

Collectively, parents teach rules, "this is just the way it is," "because I say so" and the like rather than foster self-discovery and self-determination. Ruler over the ruled. Experienced over inexperience. Powerful over the weak.

Children tend to learn from all of the people around them as well as the beliefs of the society around them. And so it is that the inquisitive child can become the blind follower. "Because mommy/daddy said so" is the mantra and we are taught to listen to our parents and that the beliefs of our caregivers are the proper beliefs. We are to believe and follow what is taught to us.

Emotional outbursts are frowned upon for their disruption rather than used as an opportunity to interpret feelings. Questioning parental ideas or authority is a nuisance at best, rather than a potential for understanding and awareness. We learn as kids to be subservient to the parental monarchy and obey the rules, "or else." Most people learn to simply follow along and I was one of those that fell in line.

This is the lens upon which we perceive the world. Our perceptions, in turn, make us form beliefs. Most of our beliefs are created when we are very young and we often aren't even aware how we came to hold these beliefs. Interestingly, these beliefs are formed before our brain is fully formed, which is why we often simply adopted the beliefs without questioning them. Even if we did question the beliefs, very few of us had the support around us to help us examine the beliefs in any serious manner. Thus, we grow up with a set of beliefs that don't even fit who we are.

We have the opportunity to change this. We can examine our beliefs and restructure them if we wish. The journey might be difficult but it is worth it. One of the best tools to use when learning how to change our beliefs and rewire our brain is self-inquiry. I detail this technique below.

SELF INQUIRY

When you read the word "self-inquiry," what arises for you? Do you think of synonyms such as self-reflection and questioning, or would you dare correlate it with the art of philosophy or metaphysics? I promise I'm not going to start quoting the likes of Aristotle's teachings to you, but it's amazing to me how many of us modern humans don't dare study the logical as well as the dreamy questioning that goes into such profound forms of inquiry. It's no wonder then that we find ourselves in the world we do. We haven't been taught to be open-minded, open-hearted questioning people.

Let's change that dynamic right now by learning how to use questions to learn about ourselves, others and the world.

On an individual level, we tend to trust our mind's automatic conclusion. Instead of challenging the soundness of our beliefs, we tend to simply believe the emotional and ego driven musings of our mind. Rather than finding a way to question from logical positions, we accept our subservience to this internal master because we rarely develop any other view of it. We always think that we are right.

Furthermore, our tendency is to accept our perceptions as fact, even though two people can be witness to the same situation and tell different stories about it. You see this in stories people tell about events that they witnessed together. Most of the time, each person tells a different story about the same event.

So indeed, we have our own truths, but truth is not fact and there can be multiple truths possible with the same facts, depending on the individual. For example, let's look at the act of smiling, one of my favorite things to do. We can see someone smiling at us and then make any number of conclusions from this. We might believe that the other person is smiling at us because they like us or that they are happy to see us. We might think that they are laughing internally at us or that they have ulterior motives. We might think that they are smiling because we reminded them of something funny. The list goes on and on. There are so many different ways to interpret a smile.

Although we know intellectually that there are many different possible reasons for any event, we typically accept what we believe as fact. We think that our perceived truth is the truth. Many of us also fall into the trap of interpreting things in a way that is detrimental to our emotional health.

We do this with many situations, acts and perceptions. It is important to question our beliefs, especially if the belief we hold is harming us. We can engage in self-inquiry to become aware of alternate possibilities.

Self-inquiry softens the mind, opens us to understanding and empathy. This helps us to move towards a sense of clarity and peace. You don't have to look all the way back to the ancient Greeks to learn this form of logical questioning. There are many modern-day teachers who focus upon this skill.

THE WORK BY BYRON KATIE

My favorite teacher on this subject is Byron Katie. She calls it "the work."

The general process goes as follows:

1. Write down or speak the thought. And when you do so, don't hold back, don't censor yourself. Give it in all it's raw emotionality.
2. Now ask yourself, "is this true?"
3. If yes, ask yourself:
   a. How do I know for certain this is true?
   b. What do I feel when I think this thought?
   c. How would I feel or who would I be without this thought?
4. One who is more practiced with self-inquiry could easily achieve great relief or enlightenment with just the above; but, many times the real proof to our entrenched thinking and limiting beliefs is proving the existence of multiple realities or possibilities.
5. As a final step, find multiple, possible truths for opposing versions of the original thought.
6. Replace in the sentence protagonist with antagonist, positive with negative, opposite action, etc. and in multiple iterations.

Katie calls this "the turnaround." According to logic, if an opposite thought was a possible truth(s), then the original supposition cannot be 100% certain. Supplying at least a couple of truths as to why opposing versions have validity can be what finally cracks the hard shell of that original thought.

AN EXAMPLE OF THE TECHNIQUE

The following is an example of a time when I used this technique in my own life. It will serve to illustrate how you can implement it in your own life.

Background story: I was in the yoga studio for class and saw a person I had gone on a date with a week earlier enter the room. The date had gone well. During the date we both mentioned we had enjoyed ourselves and that we would like to do it again. We had not spoken since so when I first saw this person enter the yoga room, it was the first contact we had. The person came into the room but didn't say anything to me. I noticed I was starting to overthink the situation so I decided to use the self inquiry technique.

1. Original thought: "This person is avoiding me and doesn't want to talk to me. They're surprised to have seen me here and now I've caught them awkwardly. They lied and the date didn't go well for them - they just said that to leave on a happy note. Ugh, I cannot trust what people say!"

2. Challenge the thought: Is this true? "Yeah, the evidence points to that. I haven't heard from them in over a week. They are not saying hello now that I'm in front of them nor acknowledging me. They're clearly avoiding me."

3. Can I know for certain? "Though it feels like all signs point to this, I guess I cannot know with absolute certainty."

4. How I feel when I believe this thought: duped, upset, ego-bruised, betrayed, ugly, etc.

5. How would I be and feel without this thought? "I would be pleased to see the person again so unexpectedly. I would be happy, hopeful and kind. I would be at peace. I would have faith that life is working out and people can be truthful."

6. The turnaround - is there any possible truth to these opposing statements to the original?

    a. I am avoiding this person and don't want to talk.

    b. I've been waiting for this person to talk to me, as I felt I had left the ball in their court at the end of the date. I don't want to be 'needy' by speaking first. I figured since I hadn't heard anything since the date, they weren't interested.

c. I don't want to talk to someone who isn't showing interest in me. I came here to enjoy this yoga class. Talking was not my goal.

d. I was uncertain how they felt about the date and thus I wasn't wholeheartedly feeling good about the date. I've been painting a rosier picture to myself.

e. This person likes me and wants to talk to me. They paid attention to me, smiled at me and engaged me in conversation during our date. They stated they really enjoyed our time together.

f. They have potentially been busy and not wanting to ask for another date when they cannot commit right now.

g. I'm shocked to see this person and am feeling awkward. When I hadn't heard from the person in over a week, I knew the possibility that they weren't interested in further dates. I figured it likely I wouldn't hear from nor see them again. I'm surprised and caught unaware by my confused feelings.

h. They aren't feeling awkward. They could have been rushing to class. They are focused on that rather than me. They could have feelings of ease and hope when they think of me. After all, I told them I had a good time on the date and would like to have another.

Story follow-up: Immediately after the class, we smiled and spoke cordially as we dressed to leave. We exchanged pleasantries as we asked one another how everything was going. We didn't bring up whether we would meet again. I wished them a good day and left.

Two weeks later, the person contacted me and asked me if they were correct in detecting 'shade' directed at them when they saw me at the yoga class. I responded, "Not at all." Before I had even seen them, I had been telling myself that if things were meant to be, they would be. It was ok if there wasn't a connection.

I would be happy with the good time I had during the date and there would be other people that I could have good dates with. I was unsure of how to deal with seeing them unexpectedly - no shade, no ill will. As the conversation continued, the person told me now that the school year was over, their schedule was opening up - they asked if I would like to meet again for further dates!

FINAL WORDS

Look at self-inquiry as the equivalent of hiring your own defense lawyer - a logical, loving version of you with your own best interests at heart. I think about this skill as the ability to question the mind's evidence, potentially rooted in patterns of trauma and blindly adopted beliefs, both conscious and unconscious. This inner lawyer challenges and creates space within our limited/rote thinking, allowing for alternative options, which allows us to let go of less empowering thinking patterns we might fall into when we drop into strangling, egotistical certainties.

Remembering to do this process takes practice, especially when we are swept up by emotion, clinging to downward spirals of negative self-talk or when we are triggered. When we do remember though and we utilize this skill, self-inquiry can help us to short-circuit our undesirable thoughts and behaviors. We can change our story mid-sentence and find freedom.

Once I started disrupting my limiting beliefs, self-deprecations, negative self-talk and emotion-driven thoughts from a place of judicious logic and self-inquiry, I found the edifice of egotistical self and dominating mind start to crumble and fall. The old uncomfortable thought patterns were exposed to the light and my mind felt more at ease. Even better, this technique has allowed my outlook for life to widen and expand, which has created wonderful opportunities for growth and transformation.

I hope you will try this amazing technique to challenge your own assumptions, perceptions and beliefs. It might just change your life.

FOOTNOTE

*When I use the word "self-inquiry," I am following what I see as a very modern, Westernized meaning. Although the yogic teachings of Ramana Maharshi's atma-vichara or vichara have correlations to the enlightenment we're going for and is a valuable practice in and of itself, it's better associated to a Western wording of "self-awareness" and is not my goal in this particular chapter. My focus here is upon the topic of questioning thoughts and assumptions that otherwise lead to unwanted behaviors, disconnection, dissatisfaction and more.

Knowing yourself is the beginning of all wisdom.

~ ARISTOTLE

ABOUT THE AUTHOR

André Roggy is a certified coach, international speaker, youth mentor, activist and writer. Being particularly passionate about the topics of conscious living, authenticity and holistic and mental health, he is eager to dialogue and promote true connections within our individual selves, amongst each other and with the world. André is currently dancing and singing to his own tune in New York City, USA.

Contact Information:
Email: aroggy@gmail.com
Linkedin: https://www.linkedin.com/in/andre-roggy

For more on Katie Byron's work, see www.thework.com

LIFESTYLE CHOICES: YOUR OUTER WORLD

Coming together is a beginning.
Keeping together is progress.
Working together is success.

~HENRY FORD

PART 5: LIFESTYLE CHOICES: YOUR OUTER WORLD

A huge part of living a healthy lifestyle is looking at all the things surrounding you that affect your life. In the last chapter we discussed your inner world, now it is time to turn to your outer world. In this section, we begin with a discussion of the importance of having healthy relationships. They say that you are the sum total of the five people you spend the most time with but in reality, you are influenced by all the people you spend time with. The people around you affect your emotional state, your spiritual state and they also influence your own beliefs about yourself which is why this aspect of life is so essential.

Next we turn to education and the need to continue to educate yourself on all the things that you need to learn to become the person you dream of being. So many adults think that their days of education are over once they grow up and this stops many people from moving towards their dreams. Let's face it, if you want to become the very best version of yourself and live your most extraordinary life, you are going to need to continually learn new things. In this fast paced world, it has become even more important than ever to be an eternal student, learning what you need to learn to become who you want to become.

Next, we move to a life purpose. This is so important and something that many people don't even think about until they are much older. As people go into their older years, they begin to wonder what their life is all about, why they were here and if their life meant anything. Why wait until you are older though? Why not think about this now? One of the greatest desires of all people is to make a difference in the world, to have a purpose, to have left the world a better place than they found it.

Finally, we end with a chapter on the importance of getting a coach. Finding the right coach to help you achieve your goals and keep you accountable might be one of the greatest things you can do for yourself. Learn about coaching and the powerful way that finding a coach might just change your life.

It's time to address our outer world. Let's go!

CHAPTER 25
IS IT WORTH IT?

by Kanika Jain

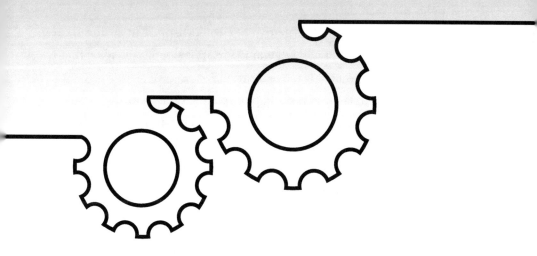

TOPIC:	Mindful living
TOOL:	Building Your Community
TECHNIQUE:	Surround yourself with people who will challenge you to be the best version of yourself. People who support and encourage you just as much as you support and encourage them.

A friend is one who knows you and loves you just the same.

~ ELBERT HUBBARD

Have you checked your friends log lately? Done a relationship audit yet? What if I tell you that our relationships and well-being are closely interrelated? Intrigued yet? If so, let me tell you a story, my story.

Years ago, I was in a toxic marriage that drained me out not only physically, but emotionally and mentally as well. The marriage was an arranged marriage and it was short. It ended in exactly nineteen days. Yes, you read that right, nineteen days.

It would seem that very little damage could happen in such a short period of time, however, I will tell you the relationship was so toxic that I suffered from the effects of it for years after.

Before my marriage, I was a happy independent working woman, with a loving family. I had a good life. I was eager to get married and start a family so I chose to go ahead with the marriage to a man I barely knew. I imagined that I was embarking on a grand adventure. I was ready to start a new life with my husband. I imagined creating a new life in a new country complete with a new house and eventually, children.

I got married and began my life in London with my new husband. The reality was totally different from what I imagined. When we reached Londonm the reality hit me so hard, like a slap in the face. My new husband was nothing like he had pretended to be, he had been wearing a façade all this time I had been getting to know him. The reality was harsh. He showed his true colors and it was not pretty.

My new husband had no time for me. He was completely cold and distant from me emotionally. He had lied about some big areas of his life such as his financial status, his job and just about everything else. For the most part, I was alone in a small dingy flat everyday. Totally alone and devoid of any human connection. The only food I had access to was red kidney beans, cereals and bananas.

My emotional condition deteriorated rapidly and my mind fogged with immense negativity As my mind clouded, my body also began to break down. I was in terrible shape. I asked to be taken to the doctor or the hospital but my husband refused. Instead, he poisoned me by giving me the wrong medication.

Thankfully, my parents were still there for me. I called them and even though I was confused and unwell, I managed to explain what was happening. After a lot of heated discussions between me, my husband and parents, it was agreed that I would fly back home to receive treatment at home with my parents. My father bought me a plane ticket and I left. I was never to see my husband again.

I don't remember the flight home much but I do remember getting to the airport and seeing my parents. I saw the look of horror on their faces as they saw me being brought off the plane in a wheelchair. They realized that I couldn't even walk, so they immediately brought me to the hospital. I was diagnosed with five different illnesses that day and was given lots of medication. I remember that I had to take ten pills per day for the next six weeks in order to make a full recovery.

This experience was one of the worst experiences of my life. I learned the hard way that one bad relationship can drastically affect your health. It was a lesson I wouldn't forget. I decided to divorce and put this chapter of my life behind me.

Although this was a terrible experience, it was also an experience which changed me completely. It was this experience that taught me the true power and real meaning of relationships. With the unconditional love and care of my family I was able to heal and come out stronger than before. I also realized how essential it is to have a supportive community around me. This was what gave me the power to change my life.

A few months after my recovery I jumped into my self-growth. I was intent upon creating a new life for myself and I knew that in order to do that, I had to learn a new way of thinking, a new way of living. I watched endless online classes and followed a lot of wellness experts. I wanted to learn everything I could.

One day, I was watching a video and I came across a platform called Mindvalley. It was a personal growth company with a record of transforming lives. I went onto the website and read story after story about the amazing growth people had experienced by using the platform. The testimonials were incredible and I was inspired by the stories I read.

I decided to join the platform right at the beginning of the global pandemic. While the world shut down and everyone retreated to their homes, I dove into the courses available on the site. It was a balm to my spirit, just what I needed. I learned how I could change my mindset and change my beliefs. I learned about the power of gratitude and forgiveness. Even more important, I learned about the power of community.

Since we were all at home, the members began to meet online. We got together and discussed what we were learning. Eventually we got to know each other really well and became friends. The platform gave me the opportunity to meet amazing beings and it has changed my life. Our deep meaningful shares, the raw vulnerabilities discussed, the immense support given, all of it was unparalleled to anything that I had experienced before. We became like a family.

They say that you are the sum total of the five people you spend the most time with. I was lucky during the pandemic to spend a lot of time with a lot more than five people. Even better, the people I met through the community were true thought leaders and changemakers. They were people who sought to become the best version of themselves. People who wanted to help make a better life for themselves and the world. I was surrounded by these amazing people and we got through the pandemic together.

When you spend a lot of time with people, it changes you. You begin to personify the qualities of the people around you. This can lead to amazing transformations if you are with the right kind of people. That's what happened for me. It happened for a lot of us.

I have learned how important it is to create a community like this around me. The greatest part of this story is that this past summer, we all met up in person for the first time and it was incredible. We had so much fun getting to know each other in real life and the best part is that we now know that the online relationships we formed are relationships we will have for the rest of our lives. I now have friends all over the world and it enhances my life to know that I can go just about anywhere and meet up with friends who are incredible people. I truly feel grateful.

BUILD YOUR COMMUNITY

Creating and being in a tribe of like-minded growth-oriented individuals is pivotal to good health. Want to know why? Let me give you some science and facts.

Social connections are shown to improve your quality of life, boost your sense of belonging and help you live longer. Community is tied to lower risk of mental health issues and even lower rates of heart disease. Strong social ties can boost your immune system and improve your emotional state. Community battles loneliness, especially in tough times..

The truth about humans is that we all need to be a part of something bigger than ourselves. Our community, connection and relationships make us feel whole and propel us forward in life so that we can live up to our full potential. The people we surround ourselves with can make our lives more meaningful, aligning us closely with our purpose in life.

Humans are emotional beings who crave love and connection. It is how we are designed. We are also tribal beings, so we thrive within groups. In fact, we have an innate fear of being kicked out of the group because in our ancient history, being kicked out of the tribe meant death. This fear is patterned into our brains.

Relationships and communities have a critical role in our lives because our relationships play a huge part in maintaining optimal health and well-being. Relationships provide emotional support, accountability, motivation, enjoyment and love. It has been found that people who have a thriving, supportive community around them live longer lives.

SInce relationships are so important, we often consciously or unconsciously keep relationships that no longer serve us. Even when a relationship is detrimental to us, we may continue it, not fully realizing the effect it is truly having on us. Toxic relationships cause feelings of low self-worth, helplessness, fear, anxiety, depression, insecurity and paranoia, to name a few. These relationships can literally ruin your mental and emotional state, which may lead to damaging physical effects.

That does not mean you walk out of every relationship which you deem unfit. Leave the ones that tear down the natural expression of who you truly are.

ACCOUNTABILITY & GOAL SETTING

Having a tribe of people who know your goals can provide a lot of motivation and accountability as you move towards your ideal life. Your friends will help to push you towards your goals and they will encourage you when you are feeling a bit unsure. The value of this cannot be overstated. A strong social group will help you move towards your goals while supporting you along the way.

Studies show that having an accountability partner makes you 65% more likely to meet your goals. This increases to 95% when you regularly check in with your partner! This support system makes your chances of success much higher than it would be if you tried to move towards your goals alone.

GREATER SUCCESS AND FULFILLMENT

True friends motivate you to work harder to reach your goals just as you help them reach theirs. When you surround yourself with people on a similar path to you, you support one another on the journey. Even better, when you surround yourself with the kind of people that inspire you, it will motivate you. Additionally, having lots of creative, intelligent friends will allow you to share skills and information. You walk together on the path and when one person finds success, they share the tips on how they got there. Success breeds more success.

YOUR NETWORK IS YOUR NET WORTH.

The more you build your network, the more you come to realize that your relationships can help you with problem solving in life challenges like work problems, career/business issues and relationships. By simply looking to your network and identifying who can help you with a problem or issue, you can focus on finding solutions rather than obsessing over the problem itself.

YOUR TRIBE AFFECTS YOUR VIBE!

The people you surround yourself with will determine how you feel. It will also serve to uplift you, inspire you and enlighten you if you have the right people around you. Assemble a tribe of people who will fill you with love, laughter and fun.

My own personal experience is nothing less than magical, I can tell you that. Today, I have my own inner circle of people who are my support system. They are there for me as much as I am there for them. They impart their wisdom and share their stories and that inspires me. My friends help me stretch and I feel bolder in my life. I am more willing to take risks and try new things. They are always there to pick me up and lift my energy when I feel low. My tribe shows me my innate potential and how to unleash it even more.

I could never imagine I would be in the position I am in today. From those days with my husband when I was at the lowest point to now, my life has totally changed. I am showered with love and care by the people around me. They want me to succeed and I want them to succeed. We walk the path together, hand in hand. I could really go on and on, but my point is a simple one:

Be with people who uplift you, who celebrate you and I can guarantee that you will see a positive trajectory of growth in your life

~ KANIKA JAIN

I have created this for myself and I want the same for you! So start right now. Look at the people around you and determine which ones uplift you and which ones don't. Spend more time with the people who uplift you and less time with the ones that make you feel depleted. And then, begin to find people who inspire you, people who are on the same path of growth and transformation as you are.

There's a Swedish proverb that I love:

Shared joy is doubled joy. Shared sorrow is half a sorrow.

BUILD YOUR TRIBE

So now that we have established that we all crave authentic connections constantly, the question is how to go about meeting those golden gems and building long-lasting, meaningful friendships and communities?

The answer is very easy- be intentional about meeting new people.

You can find them when you make a genuine attempt of taking the time out to look for them. The first step is to get really clear on what you are looking for in a relationship. Turn inward and determine what your core values and attributes are.

Then, get clear on the kind of people you hope to attract with these specific questions.

Ask yourself:

- What are the qualities, characteristics, values of those who are in your circle?
- Do they connect with your core values?
- Do they reflect on who you are now as well as who you are becoming?
- Spot those people who no longer match your attributes and values and fade them out of your circle.

- These questions will serve as the building blocks of your inner circle formation.

Once you have clarity on this crucial piece, you can then go out and find those real connections.

Some simple tips include:

- Go online and check the local communities to join that have similar attributes to yours.
- Start a conversation- Give someone a call or write or email them and let them know how you feel.
- Join and support voluntary organizations matching your values.
- Have family meals to foster and celebrate your achievements, life lessons or stories of the day. Parents may want to include younger children to nurture the importance of connection at an early age.
- Blog it out- sharing your views and values on online platforms.
- Hold online masterminds with like-minded individuals which is an exclusive space to track your progress, commemorate your accomplishments and hold the space for your honest shares, or ask for help.
- Go for coffee dates or kayaking trips with friends if that stirs you.

The list is endless. However, a key point to note is to "Rinse and repeat the above steps every six months" as you may want to elevate to a different circle as you grow.

SELF LOVE

Another key area mostly overlooked is your relationship with yourself. Your relationship with yourself is crucial for overall health and well-being. Self-love and care nourish you and help keep your energy levels strong.

What exactly is self-love? Simply put, self-love is catering to your inner needs and in doing so, developing and evolving into the person you strive to be. The more you practice self love, the more you appreciate yourself. Soon you will learn to celebrate your inner beauty and wisdom and you will come to respect the core of your being. This helps you to develop a solidified sense of who you truly are. In a nutshell, you become your own "Forever Cheerleader."

Self-care builds not only your self-worth and emotional resilience, but also boosts your productivity, increases your success, creates a sense of joy, helps you feel fulfilled and enhances your desire to live your life's purpose.

Putting yourself first is not an easy decision, especially when you are responsible for others' well-being in different capacities. Learn to change your beliefs around self care and remember that you are at your best when you are feeling your best. Taking care of yourself is a great way to give yourself the time and space to create a life where you are able to take care of others.

Having time for yourself does not mean you are pushing others away. The truth is, a lot of us find ourselves in this trap, including me. I feel guilty when I decide to do things for myself. I always feel like "I should be helping someone else." However counterintuitive it may sound, the reality is that taking care of yourself will help you see the value in your relationships, rather than see them as a chore. You cannot give something you don't have, so give yourself the love you need so you have the bandwidth to give others this same level of love. Come from a place of filling yourself with love first so that you can automatically overflow the rest to the others.

So, my beautiful one, embody the expression of self-love in your own unique ways.

SELF CARE TIPS

- Be aware of your negative thoughts and talk positively to yourself.
- Use positive affirmations, like 'I Am Enough', 'I Am Strong', 'I Am Beautiful', 'My Life is Wonderful' are very helpful in this area. A whole list of positive affirmations is available on the internet if you just search for it.

- Personal tip: Keep 4-5 affirmations as reminders on your mobile to pop up on different time slots daily so that you read them and feel motivated.
- Use the power of "No" and honor yourself.
  - Start saying "No" to things that don't align with your values and beliefs.
- Ditch the comparison to others and work on honing your strengths.
- Ask for help when you need to, as a lot of us always think that we can do it all by ourselves.
- Do 1 thing you love daily like reading a book, dancing to music, cooking, etc.
- Meditate in any form.
- Reflect and introspect ask yourself-
  - What worked well today?
  - What is to be improved?
  - What am I grateful for?
  - What magic did I witness today?
- Have a spa date to just pamper yourself, or take an afternoon nap to rejuvenate yourself.
- Stand in front of the mirror, look into your eyes (focus on the left eye) and keep repeating "I Love Myself" gently for five minutes.
  - If five minutes feels too long, begin with one minute and work your way up to five.
- Put yourself at the top of your to do list every single day and witness the rest fall into place. Trust me, you will thank yourself later. The time I give to myself is a part of my *daily* self-care routine and it is non-negotiable!

Today I take pride in loving myself like there is no tomorrow. I also have a battalion of superbly amazing changemakers as my dear friends, who not only celebrate me and my success but embrace my low points and failures as well. These people give me solid personal advice and tips. I always say "We are not self-made but community-made."

Take the time to create deep, true relationships with yourself and others. Once you do this, you will find respect, love, appreciation and belonging with others.

FINAL WORDS

So here's your reminder- Go ahead, love yourself, start now. Then, seek out people who are doing their inner work too. Lean on the people in your life for support. Offer your unique gifts to the people around you. Move beyond the surface level.

Whenever you feel in doubt about a connection, ask yourself- is it worth it and aligned to me truly? Heeding to this one question and answering it truthfully from your heart could be a game changer for you. You will be astounded to see how happy your life can become.

I firmly believe that *you* and only *you* are the creator of your life. So go create.

Find your inner beauty and then find a community with the spirit you align with. It's waiting for you with open arms to be embraced and the shift within you will be instantaneous, I promise. You just need to believe in it and be open to it.

If you want to learn more about self love, read this book, it's one of my favorites: *Love Yourself Like Your Life Depends On It* by Kamal Ravikant.

I leave you with this to ponder:

> *But we can contribute to the schism, or we can*
> *be a balm of kindness and goodness,*
> *and look to bring love, light, illumination,*
> *presence, connectedness.*
> *It's amazing how that can shift another's world.*

I know what it feels like for me to receive that.
I know what it feels like to offer that
and I think that's a beautiful reality that
sometimes in the busyness of life,
we can forget how impactful in a
moment we can touch another,
we can reach another, we can move
another, we can remind each other
because we're mirroring each other and as we're offering that
we're experiencing that ourselves. We're all reflecting each other.

~ SAGE ROBBINS

I absolutely love connecting with like minded people. Please reach out to share your stories as you embark upon your journey to build your tribe. I would love to hear from you.

In love and community,
Kanika

ABOUT THE AUTHOR

Kanika Jain is a Holistic Health Coach, Quantum Healer, Quantum Flow Practitioner & Chartered Financial Analyst (CFA).

She loves to empower people to know and love themselves, equipping them with tools to live meaningful & radiant lives, propelling them to realize their own inner power to "evolve consciously and authentically".

Contact Information:
Email: kanika.j6@gmail.com
Instagram: kanikajain.love
Facebook: https://www.facebook.com/kanika.jain.92317

Always walk through life as if you have something new to learn and you will.

~Vernon Howard

I find that the harder I work, the
more luck I seem to have.

~Thomas Jefferson

CHAPTER 26

EDUCATION AND CONSISTENCY

by Ashutosh Khemka

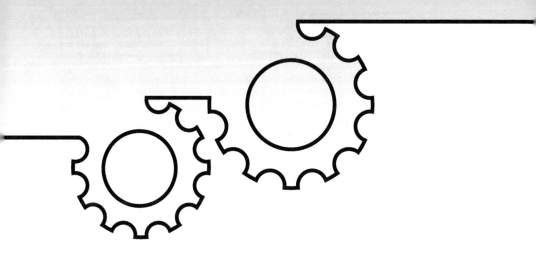

TOPIC:	Self Motivation
TOOL:	Consistency
TECHNIQUE:	Create a system of learning where you constantly improve yourself. Use your knowledge to create healthy habits that will move you towards the life you dream of.

*It is on us whether we let opportunities ride us
on top or allow challenges to drown us.
The choice is always ours.*

~ASHUTOSH KHEMKA

My life before I learned about biohacking was miserable. I always felt a lack of energy, low mood and I had very little motivation. I had lost my self esteem and I felt mentally, physically and spiritually broken. I had lost all direction.

When I saw myself in the mirror I always cursed myself for not taking care of myself. I wished I were someone else. I lost all interest in my appearance. I didn't even want to buy new clothing because nothing fit me well. I wanted to flush my old life and start over. I knew I had to do something but I wasn't sure what to do. I had a vague notion that I had to dive deep and explore who I really was, but I didn't know when to start.

During this bad phase of my life, I was not able to find a reason to change. I wanted to uplift and create a new life for myself, but the motivation was not there.

Then, my son was born. The birth of my son was like a sign from the universe, giving me the signal I needed. I understood how important it was for me to regain my zest for life, my vigor and especially, my health. I knew I wanted to be the best dad I could possibly be and in order to that, I had to be in peak physical, mental and emotional shape. I wanted to change myself for my son. My child made me want to be a better man.

I knew that I had to listen to the message I was receiving. I wanted my son to grow up to be proud that I was his dad. I wanted to inspire him to be the best he could be so I made a solemn promise to myself and him that I would do whatever it took to push to become the best version of myself. I wanted to achieve the highest level of health for myself and my family.

But where to begin?

I decided it was best to start with strength training. I began to notice changes in my body and I was happy to see that I was very quickly able to see the results of my efforts. This gave me the motivation to do even more, so I started to eat right and nourish my body the way it needed for optimal health. These were small changes at first but with each success, I was able to celebrate my win and that kept my energy high. I continued making lifestyle changes and I began to lead a very disciplined life, which made me feel super energized.

It was not just the changes I had made to my diet and exercise routine that helped me. Instead, what really worked for me was showing up regularly for myself. It was the consistency that was yielding my results. The consistency was the powerful tool that drove my transformation.

Now I am in a completely different place from where I started. I have achieved my initial goal of losing 25 pounds (11 kilos) and I look great. My muscles are developing well and I am fully shredded now. I am proud of my body and will continue to increase my muscle strength and shape. I am now taking it up a notch with a six month total transformation challenge. I am excited to see where I will be at the end of the six months.

This was my journey and I would like to share the steps I took so that you can go on your own journey. Finding the motivation you need will help you along the journey, so before you even begin find something that will serve to motivate you to stick to your plan to become the best version of yourself.

Once you have your motivation, your why, it's time to set some goals. It is essential to plan our goals first in order to know where we are going. Having goals provides the blueprint, the directions you need to make the journey a little easier.

Once you have your goals, set a plan. It might be helpful to look for mentors to help you along the way. One thing which I have experienced is that you will never get all the answers from one mentor. You need to have different mentors. For instance, you can have one physical mentor to train you on a daily basis, but then you can use books, podcasts and videos as your secondary mentor to find all the important answers of your life. Think about what resources you will use as you begin your transformation of body, mind and spirit.

Are you ready? Let's go!

FOUR IMPORTANT PERSPECTIVES

There are four important perspectives which can help you create smart, effective change into your life. They are education and having a mentor, consistency and patience in the processes, having an end goal in mind and focusing on your habits. Let's look at each in turn.

EDUCATION AND MENTORS

Education is the key to all change. There has never been an easier time to get the information you need to create the change you seek in your life. You can find anything you need to learn by searching the internet. You can listen to podcasts, read articles, watch videos or do an online course. You can also read books and find teachers who will help you to improve the area of your life you want to improve.

You can begin by learning about nutrition and what kinds of foods will nourish your body best. Pay attention as you eat so you can learn which foods work best for your body. Learn about the importance of hydration and figure out how much water you need to drink each day to stay hydrated. Learn about the different strength and cardiovascular exercises there are and incorporate them into your life. Create a learning plan for yourself, detailing what you want to learn in the days, weeks and years ahead.

It is also nice to find mentors who will guide you as you begin to make changes to your lifestyle. Seek out teachers who inspire you and learn from them. Go to weekend retreats and workshops so that you can meet like-minded people who are on the same path. This is a great way to find mentors that will help you on your journey. It is also a great way to find some accountability partners who you can check in with to keep your motivation high.

Allow learning to be a part of your daily routine and find mentors, teachers and friends who will support you on your journey.

CONSISTENCY AND PATIENCE

Consistency and patience are two important tools that will help you to continue to stick with your plan as you make your way towards achieving your goals.

The Merriam Webster dictionary defines consistency as "marked by harmony, regularity or steady continuity." This means showing up daily and achieving smaller wins each day. These minor wins will add up over time and eventually, you will reach bigger milestones.

Patience is also important because the changes may not be obvious in the beginning. It's easy to give up when you don't see results quickly. You might lose your rhythm when you don't see much change and this might lead you to falsely believe that the process doesn't work. Having patience allows you to keep with it even when it gets tough. I remember that it took me a full year to lose 25 pounds. It was frustrating in the beginning, especially because when I changed my eating habits, I didn't see the results for a few months. I had to be patient and stay committed, consistently sticking with my plan until eventually, I did see the change.

So use consistency and patience as you create new habits. Remember, our old habits are not easy to break, so it is essential to keep your eyes on the goal. Do not get into the trap of giving up. Stick with it and you will see changes. Trust the process, be patient, show up daily and you will have a transformative change for sure.

KEEP THE END GOAL IN MIND

It is important to have clarity around the goals you want to accomplish. You have to visualize yourself as the person you want to become so that you can keep your end goal in mind. When you have an end goal, your mind actually begins to search for the information it needs to get you there. This helps you to progress quickly. Remember, when you set a goal for yourself, your mind prepares your body to work in that direction.

When I decided to become healthy, I had a very clear goal in mind. I knew I wanted to lose weight and I set targets for where I wanted to be at the end of each month. I decided to give myself a year to lose the weight, so my monthly targets were achievable and I hit them each month. Each time I reached my target, I would celebrate myself. There were even some challenges along the way, like when I got injured and had to be on bed rest, but I weathered the challenge. I was back on track in two months because I had trained my mind to work towards my goal. Having the end goal in mind was an essential part of my journey.

FOCUS ON YOUR HABITS

Our habits give the framework for our success. They are the building blocks for our transformation.

Begin by building effective habits throughout your day. You can create a morning routine and an evening routine, which will help you begin and end your days in a calm and peaceful way. Schedule time each day where you will fit in exercise, meal times, time with loved ones and time to just relax.

When you schedule your time, you will become more productive. Use your habits as a way to keep a structure and format to your life. Your habits will ultimately determine the quality of life, so be mindful as you add habits into your day. Start with one habit and once that is established, add another habit. Slowly, over time, you will create a day filled with healthy habits that support you in moving towards your best life.

FINAL WORDS

Education and mentors, consistency and patience, keeping the end goal in mind and creating healthy habits are the four foundational principles upon which you will build your new life. Keeping these principles in mind will give you the results you wanted and will also help you to become a better person. You will build your strength and your character so that you can achieve anything that you want in your life.

It is my hope that you go on a journey of self discovery and self motivation so that you can begin to construct the life you dream of. You deserve it.

Please feel free to reach out to me. I would love to hear your stories.

With Respect and Motivation,
Ashutosh

People never learn anything by being told,
they have to find out for themselves.

~ P A U L O C O E L H O

ABOUT THE AUTHOR

Ashutosh is a firm believer in tuning into the melody of life. He believes that we need to play different strings on guitar to make good music and similarly that in order to become superhuman, we have to walk on a path of self discovery. Along the way there will be all sorts of experiences but the journey will make you stronger physically, mentally and emotionally.

Ashutosh approaches health from a holistic viewpoint. He advocates for taking full responsibility for your situation in life, to look for things to be grateful for and then to roll up your sleeves to get to work.

Ashutosh believes that one of the keys to transformation is practicing self love. This was the way that he was able to fight the battle and conquer his negative behaviors. He helps people to have a winning mindset in order to reach the heights they hope to reach.

Contact Information:
ashutosh.khemkaa@gmail.com
Author's website: https://linktr.ee/kidikools
LinkedIn - https://www.linkedin.com/in/ashutosh-khemka-29051a14/

**When a person can't find a deep sense of meaning,
they distract themselves with pleasure.**

~Viktor E. Frankl

**A journal is a self-empowering, self-realizing map
we create for ourselves to better our lives.**

~Andrew Pacholy

CHAPTER 27
LIFE PURPOSE
by Kunihiro Matsuo

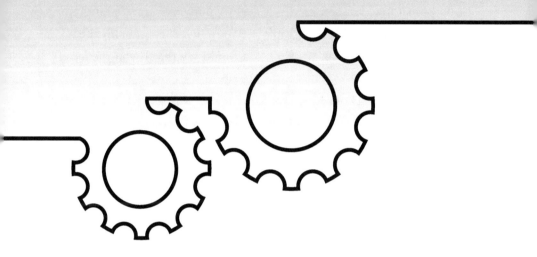

TOPIC: Finding Your Life Purpose

TOOL: Journaling and the Ten Basic Human Needs

TECHNIQUE: Go on a journey of self discovery so that you can discover who you really are and what you really want.

You were put on this earth to achieve your greatest self, to live out your purpose and to do it courageously.

~ STEVE MARABOLI

As I open my mouth, a spoonful of tasty cereal enters, as my grandmother feeds me a mouthful of love. Throughout my childhood, I was constantly surrounded by love. My mother and father, my two grandmothers, a nanny and a maid were always present.

I was born in Santa Monica, Los Angeles and raised in Beverly Hills. I'm not going to lie, my childhood memories were awesome. I was blessed to be born the eldest son of the Matsuo Family. My great-grandfather built a family foundation, which allowed me to live the rest of my life with money and time freedom. Most people would say that I won the lottery ticket of life.

My grades in school were good, my future was set. I knew I would grow up and take over the family foundation so I had very little stress in my life. I applied and got accepted to the University of California in 2007. My university life was beautiful, since I did not need to study as my future was already assured. This allowed me to party instead for the four years I was there.

In 2015, my father asked me to apply to a Master's program in Europe which he believed would benefit the family business in the future. I agreed. To me, it was simply another occasion to party!

At the time, Jordan Belfort, the main character in *Wolf of Wall Street* was my hero. With that in mind, I set off for Europe at the age of 26 in 2015 to become Jordan Belfort and I absolutely nailed it. I partied, experimented with drugs and lived the "YOLO" life. I had the freedom to do whatever I desired in my life. I was young, I was money rich and I was time rich. But was I a happy man?

Well, I will say that my four years of university and my years in Europe getting my Masters degree were very fun. I would say I was pretty happy. However, I still had too much time on my hands. I found that I had no idea how to spend abundant time available to me before I was to take over the family business. I felt lost in life to be honest.

Fortunately, journaling discovered me. In May of 2017, I was inspired by a new incoming employee who joined one of my father's companies.

He was very young and radiated enthusiasm and clarity. I was naturally drawn to him and curious of his secret.

I asked him, "Why are you so full of enthusiasm and energy?"

He told me his secret was journaling, so I decided to try it out. I began to journal daily and slowly, over time, it began to transform my life.

Journaling changed my life and it can change yours too. Let's look closely at what journaling is and why you should try it.

JOURNALING

What is journaling?

Journaling is a simple process where you sit and write about whatever comes to mind. You can journal about your day, about issues or challenges you are facing or about decisions you need to make. You can use a typical journal style book or you can use an online document to write your thoughts. You can journal daily or take a few minutes throughout the day to jot down what is coming up for you.

Why Should You Journal?

Journaling is an essential habit that helps you to live a fulfilling life, because it allows you to create a relationship with yourself. People don't realize how much they don't really know themselves. Most of us have no clue of who we are and what we want to do in life. Most of humanity is plugged into the matrix and controlled by the system. We are asleep to our deepest desires and unaware of what brings us joy. And yes, that included me back then.

How to Journal

When I began journaling in 2017, the format was very simple. I used journaling prompts, which I answered every night. I made sure to print out the journaling template so that I could fill it out by hand. I found that writing on paper is more intimate than typing since it is tangible. I highly recommend writing over typing since you can memorize what you write more than what you type.

The five main questions I answered at night were

1. What were some things that went well today?
2. What did I learn today?
3. If I could relive today, what would I have done differently?
4. What am I grateful for today?
5. What are three goals I plan to achieve tomorrow?

I also had a column on the left side of the paper where I put in the time schedule of the plan for the following day.

How to Start Journaling

If you are a beginner to journaling, I recommend you begin with these five simple questions to get into the habit of journaling. If there are too many questions, it can get overwhelming.

When I began, it wasn't easy to continue this habit every day and there were times where I didn't journal for weeks because I didn't want to confront myself. I always went back to it though and eventually it became a habit. It does take practice and patience to continue, so be kind to yourself as you begin to create the journaling habit.

How Journaling Helped Me

Ever since graduating university in 2011, I was unsuccessful in finding a life partner and felt extremely lonely. I spent a lot of years hating myself, to be honest. Journaling helped me to get to the bottom of my feelings about myself and about my life.

Once I had been journaling for a year, I met my current life partner who I married in 2019. I truly believe journaling allowed me to manifest this reality. Journaling gave me direction in life. It gave me clarity about who I was and what I wanted.

The act of answering the five journaling prompts every day helped me to change my mindset. It helped me to practice positive thinking and gratitude daily. The act of choosing their goals to accomplish each day was also critical to my transformation. I picked different goals, but I noticed that over time, my goals became much more conducive to living a fabulous life. I started with goals like, "don't get hung over" or "hit on three girls tonight and get their numbers" and moved to goals like, "get up early," "initiate a new project at work" and "work out each day."

Having to write my goals down each day gave me new direction in life. Meeting my life partner brought more joy and happiness into my life. Now I had money, time and a partner. However, there was still something missing in my life. I didn't feel fulfilled. I wasn't truly happy yet. I continued to party and experiment with new drugs because I wanted to fill this huge void in my heart. So, I naturally made it a mission to seek happiness.

MY PERSONAL TRANSFORMATION

I began to study personal transformation and I began to consume everything I could find. I dove into this world with enthusiasm and excitement. I found a lot of great content online, but one of the best things I found was an educational company called Mindvalley. I really enjoyed their content and was learning quickly. I decided to attend a live event hosted by the company called A-fest and it blew my mind.

The experience caused a paradigm shift. I got this absolute "knowing" that there exists a spiritual world out there and what brings meaning and happiness to life was having a life's purpose. I became obsessed with my life's purpose.

Pursuing my life's purpose was very interesting. Most people strive for financial freedom, so they don't have to work anymore and so they have the freedom to travel around the world freely. Since I had been born with all the freedom, money and time I could want but was not happy or fulfilled, I knew there had to be something more. I am grateful that I was able to realize that money, possessions or lifestyle cannot make you happy. It helped me to understand that finding my life purpose was the key to fill this void in my heart.

Okay, so my job was to find my life purpose, but as many of you may expect, it wasn't that easy. I felt seriously lost in life and continued to consume even more drugs to feel alive. I distracted myself, telling myself that partying was my life purpose. I did exactly what Viktor Frankly said, "When a person can't find a deep sense of meaning, they distract themselves with pleasure." I got into trouble with the authorities. I got sick for a while.

I needed help.

Fortunately, despite feeling so low, I had the support and love from my family and friends, so I was able to pull myself together and not give up on myself. I wanted to find my life's purpose, I wanted to find happiness.

In the end of 2021, I finally found a mentor in life who guided and coached me to finally discover what it means to live a Life of Purpose! I am confident to say that there is no correct answer to what the purpose of life is, but for the rest of this chapter I will share with you my belief on life purpose and how to fulfill it.

My intention is to help you find the most meaningful and happiest life you deserve to live. After 33 years of my life seeking happiness, this is the recipe that is working for me now.

So, before I share the tools, I'd like to clarify my current definition of My Life Purpose.

MY LIFE PURPOSE

My Life Purpose is to "Experience the most Happiness I possibly can within this Body".

Firstly, it is essential to clarify your own definition of Happiness. Honestly, no one ever agrees with the definition of happiness and never probably will. All the famous philosophers in history never agreed with one concept. But thanks to my mentor, I came up with my own definition of happiness that resonates with me today.

TEN BASIC NEEDS

Have you heard of Maslow's Hierarchy of Needs? My mentor upgraded this pyramid and discovered there are ten Basic Human Needs. All of humanity feels happy when these ten basic human needs are met. So, my definition of the Purpose of Life is to satisfy all these ten basic human needs as much as you can within this lifetime by creating habits and systems to do so.

The key is to work from the bottom of the pyramid and work your way to the top. If the needs on the bottom of the pyramid are not met, the whole pyramid crumbles, so it is essential to work from the bottom for long-term and sustainable happiness.

Use your journal to keep track of your progress as you make your way through the ten basic human needs. Write down your thoughts on the area you are working on, ideas for improvement and note your successes as you continue to move through the pyramid.

The Ten Basic Human Needs from the Bottom to Top

1. Physiological Needs: Health, Breathing, Water, Sleep, Food
2. Safety Needs: Shelter, Health, Security
3. Love / Belonging: Family, Friendship
4. Acceptance: Feeling of Being Accepted (by yourself and others)

5. Growth: Becoming Better, Learning
6. Power: Self-Esteem, Confidence, Money, Achievement
7. Freedom: Financial Freedom, Mental Freedom
8. Fun: Pleasure, Play, Life Experiences
9. Self-Actualization: Achieving your Dreams, Achieving Full Potential
10. Transcendence: Contribution, Legacy, Service, Joy

People have different tastes and preferences, so people feel happier when one need is met than another, but we can all agree that we all feel happy when these needs are met.

The Dalai Lama says the purpose of life is to be happy, which I define as satisfying these ten needs. So here are my ten personal habits. For each section you can begin today to journal about each of them where you determine where you are and then you create a plan to move towards goals that will satisfy these ten basic human needs.

Physiological Health

I have a feeling many of us know health is important and are already creating habits and routines to satisfy this need. Let me bring a different lens to the picture. The top three priorities for health in order are breathing, water and sleep.

Why? Because it is said that you can't survive three minutes without breathing, three days without water and ten days without sleep.

Maximize the satisfaction of these needs through your daily routines.

Breathing: Make sure to do your breathing exercises every morning.
Water: Drink the best water (Kangen Water).
Sleep: Get some sunlight in the morning to release serotonin.

Safety Needs

Fortunately, our safety needs are usually met if you are living in a developed country. It is said it takes three hours before you die in a harsh environment (extreme heat or cold) so make it a habit to avoid extreme heat and cold environments.

Love / Belonging

The most important skill required to build strong human connection is "communications skills". Steven Covey's Habit #5 is essential: "First Seek to Understand, Then to Be Understood." Most of us fail at communicating because we are so busy trying to be understood by the other person.

Make it a priority to fully understand the other person.

Ask questions for clarity. Repeat what the other person says.

Acceptance

The habit I recommend here is to accept all the emotions you are experiencing without judging them or yourself. We often judge ourselves for feeling sad, mad, jealous, etc.

We even judge ourselves for judging ourselves.

We must understand that there are no "positive" or "negative" emotions. Sadness, anger and jealousy are beautiful emotions that paint a picture of the human experience. They are information for us, they point us to where we need to do some work.

The technique here is to practice "feeling" our emotions instead of labeling or judging them. Emotions are said to only last 90 seconds. If you still feel angry after 90 seconds, you are just recreating the story in your head, so stop thinking and feel it in your body fully. Bring your awareness to the body sensations of the emotion.

Growth

The number one habit here is to be a lifelong student. Be curious and learn the things that will help you become a better person. To really set in the lessons, make sure that you teach what you learn to someone as soon as possible. If you can't teach what you learn, you don't know it. You retain 90% of what you learn if you can teach it, so make it a habit of teaching something you just learned.

Power

To feel powerful, make it a habit to choose and use empowering words. Use conscious language.

Did you know, our subconscious mind does not recognize "subjects"? Therefore, if you call someone "stupid", you are basically calling yourself stupid as well. Whatever word you use, it affects your self-esteem, so choosing words to elevate your self-esteem is crucial. The words you use create your reality.

Freedom

True freedom is the freedom of choice. No one can take away your freedom of choice. You always have a choice. You are where you are today because of all the choices you made.

Make it a habit to say "I choose to…"

Even if you decide to play victim or make excuses, say "I choose to play victim or I choose to make excuses."

An empowering statement is "I choose to live a life of purpose." Try repeating that to yourself a few times a day. It will change the way you think.

Fun

We all have the ability to create "fun" in everything we do.

Look at children, they can create fun out of anything. They can move a toy car back and forth for hours. Take a lesson and find what is fun for you.

The key to happiness is to make it a habit to find the fun in everything you do. Before doing any task, make it a habit to ask yourself, "How can I have more fun doing this task?" We all have this ability, we just forgot about it as we grew up.

Self-Actualization

This is Steven Covey's Habit #2 "Begin with the End in Mind".

If you want to manifest your goals, simply determine what goal you desire to manifest and work backwards. Make it a habit of doing so, whether it's a three year goal or a daily goal. Always begin with the end in mind.

Self-Transcendence

The most powerful habit you can do every day and change the world is to smile at another soul. I am serious.

After creating this habit, I noticed a huge change in my life. Each time my eyes meet the eyes of another and I smile, I feel fulfilled. It is amazing how your smile can lighten up another soul. You'll be surprised how much happiness this brings to your life. All this time, I was unhappy and unfulfilled partying and wasting all that money, when a simple smile lightening up another soul brought me so much joy.

Happiness to me is satisfying these ten basic human needs. The amazing part is you don't need to be rich to do so. All you need to do is to examine each area and then journal until you fully understand where you are and where you want to go.

Life is actually very simple.

Keep satisfying these ten basic human needs by creating habits and systems and continue to make the foundation of the pyramid bigger and bigger.

We are each given a different life purpose. The purpose of life is to find out your life purpose and then to live it.

You know you are living your life purpose when you

- feel excited all the time with everything you do
- feel energized and inspired
- feel joy making other people happy in your own divine way

It is my life mission to help as many souls as possible to live their life purpose. I believe it is everyone's life mission to do the same.

When you live your life purpose, you allow others to do so as well.

With Lots of Smiles and Love,
Kunihiro

The best way to lengthen out our days is to walk steadily and with a purpose.

~ CHARLES DICKENS

ABOUT THE AUTHOR

Kunihiro Matsuo was born in Santa Monica, Los Angeles and raised in Tokyo, Japan. Though being born to a wealthy family, he gradually realized that having money, time and freedom did not bring him true happiness.

After realizing this, he began seeking what true happiness was and discovered that a Life of Purpose was what brought him true happiness.

Today, he uses his wide experience and wisdom to bring light to people to pursue a truly happy and fulfilling life everyone deserves and desires to live.

Together with his lifetime partner, Rin, he is building the Jiaiii Community. This is a community with a mission to liberate as many souls as possible. The motto is "You can Have it All."

Contact Information:
Instagram: @jiaiii_hiro

Your anger? It's telling you where you feel powerless.
Your anxiety? It's telling you that
something in your life is off balance.
Your fear? It's telling you what you care about.
Your apathy? It's telling you where you're
overextended and burnt out.
Your feelings aren't random, they are messengers.
And if you want to get anywhere,
you need to be able to let them speak to
you and tell you what you really need.

~Brianna Weist

CHAPTER 28

COACHING: THE SECRET SAUCE OF EXTRAORDINARY LIVING

by Karen Stanton

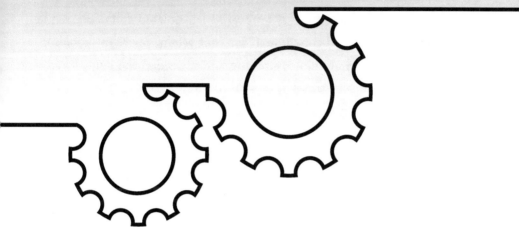

TOPIC:	Transforming Your Life
TOOL:	Coaching
TECHNIQUE:	Find a coach who will help you clarify your goals and supercharge your life.

Never react emotionally to criticism.
Analyze yourself to determine whether it is justified.
If it is, correct yourself. Otherwise, go on about your business.

~ NORMAN VINCENT PEALE

My life today is amazing. I am in great health, I look good, I feel good and I have a true sense of purpose. I love my job as a coach who helps people transform their lives. I have a wonderful group of friends and associates who support me, encourage me and motivate me to be the best person I can be. In short, my life is great.

It wasn't always like this.

Years ago, I went through a very difficult time. My marriage had broken up and after my divorce, I moved. I felt isolated and depressed. My health was at an all-time low. I was overweight, obese in fact and I felt terrible. I did not enjoy exercising and I avoided the gym. I had an aversion to the very thought of walking into a gym as a matter of fact. I was not eating well, I was not exercising and my physical state was not good.

I decided to get a coach because I really didn't know where to turn. Through coaching I became more aware of my unhealthy habits and de-cided to dedicate myself to becoming healthy. I made a promise to myself that I would learn what I needed to learn to turn my life around.

I began to study fitness and came across a great program called 10X Fitness. I loved the course because it had a lot of scientific evidence that helped me to learn about my body. I learned how my body worked an-atomically and physically through the detailed and easy-to-understand diagrams. I gained a new understanding of longevity and morbidity. This was enough for me to finally make the connections that I needed to have a huge mindset shift. I decided to dive deep into the world of fitness.

Although I had this massive mindset shift, I still had a lot of resistance to overcome. I was determined to succeed, even as I struggled for months to learn a new way of being. I was working with my coach to create a new identity for myself, one that would empower me and help me to sustain these new healthy habits that I was incorporating into my life. This was a paradigm shift for me.

I was learning to take responsibility for myself and to care for myself. I was moving into a new vision for who I was. I was creating an identity that embodied health and wellness. This new identity helped me to install the maintenance routines required for me to stay healthy.

Internal shifts allowed me to see the change I wanted. I made goals to create the change I desired. I made a plan to release 26 pounds even though that seemed difficult at the time. I resolved to do it. I decided I wanted to improve other health markers too and set goals to reduce my blood pressure, cholesterol and fat percentages. I wanted to improve my bone density as well. I also wanted to reduce my stress and become more peaceful, calm and serene.

I saw the outcome of who I wanted to be. I believed in this new version of myself so much that I even saw that vision when I looked in the mirror. I was creating a new identity that I believed in. I didn't hope that I would be able to become that person, I knew I would be able to become that person.

My coach explained to me that in order to create the change I wanted, I had to tie the goals to something that motivated me, that inspired me. I thought about it and realized that I wanted to do this for myself but even more, I wanted to do it so that I could inspire others. I decided that I would become healthy and happy and then I would become a coach to help others do the same. This became my mission, my life's purpose. It was my desire to serve others that gave me the motivation I needed.

Anytime I faced obstacles, anytime I felt like I was getting nowhere, I leaned on this vision of being a coach. It gave me the passion and drive I needed to keep going. This was one of the keys.

I worked with various coaches throughout the process. I got help when I felt stalled or when I needed expert guidance. This was the best thing I could have done. My coaches were the secret to my success. I honor them because I know I couldn't have done it without them.

I have now made the transition into living a lifestyle that empowers me. I have taken control of all aspects of my life and I love it. I expect this healthy lifestyle to continue as long as I live. I *know* this lifestyle will continue as long as I live.

Are you a person who's decided you want a healthier and more abundant lifestyle? If so, keep reading, I'll show you the way.

COACHING

There are so many programs, tools, books and classes out there. If you've spent money, bought foods or supplements or gym memberships or exercise gadgets, started excitedly and then months or years later found yourself right back where you started, you aren't alone. I did that for years.

I discovered many tools and techniques that can help people achieve their health and wellness goals, but there was a secret ingredient that I was missing. Once I added that to the systems I chose to apply, I got results that thrilled me.

The secret ingredient is not so secret and I will share it with you.

It's coaching.

You might be surprised that corporations, including many of the biggest and most successful ones, hire coaches to help them achieve goals and solve problems. Businesses all over the world hire coaches to expand their business, to support their executives and to provide professional development for their management teams.

Who else has a coach or several coaches?

Top athletes, actors, musicians and singers and leaders in every sphere of life. People who are serious about the results they want turn to coaches.

And you can too.

Coaching is a transformational process. It is a self-empowering tool that enables you to move from pain and limitations to a much happier, healthier lifestyle.

Coaches can help you shift your perspective and shift your identity. They will provide the structure and support you need as you begin to change your life. Coaches can guide you to learn what you need to in order to get where you want to go. Coaches are great because they allow you to dive deep to discover how you got where you are today and they also help you figure out where you want to go tomorrow. Even better, really good coaches will help you create a framework for transformation.

Transformation is the process by which you can achieve goals and move towards the healthier and more abundant lifestyle you desire. Coaches empower through a process as thinking partners.

There are many different types of coaches including health coaches, life coaches, business coaches, holistic coaches, divorce coaches, spiritual coaches and relationship coaches to name a few.

Coaches can help guide you through a host of problems including but not limited to: stress, overwhelm, toxic environments, obesity, health concerns, work-life balance and lifestyle design.

There is a coach for everything and the great thing about coaches is that most of them are results oriented. Instead of constantly talking about the problems and issues of the past, they help you put the past into perspective so that you can focus on the future. Coaches provide a safe space where you can define your purpose and values and create goals and desires to ensure you feel aligned with your core values.

A coach is an objective, impartial champion who creates a unique space to explore opportunities. A coach will listen to you and help you recognize your own strength and resilience. They will help you to examine your behaviors, beliefs, choices and decisions so that you can use this information to create change in your life.

Coaches help you organize your thoughts by asking open-ended questions, reflecting on your current thoughts and beliefs and shining a light on behaviors, new decisions and choices you can make. Your coach might support you by brainstorming, helping you find information and providing referrals to other professionals, research studies and specialized training.

Even though I wanted changes in my life and fitness, I stayed stuck in familiar and comfortable behaviors for many years. Even though I was unhealthy and didn't feel or look well, I stayed stuck in my old patterns.

This is because it is always easier to stay with what we know than what we don't know. One of the primary functions of the brain is to keep you alive and resist what is unfamiliar. Returning to what is familiar is your brain's strategy for keeping you alive. This is why change is so hard. It is not impossible, though. We can retrain our brains to embrace change. It takes effort, but the effort is well worth it.

Coaching is a methodology that can assist in self-discovery, so that you can develop new sustainable habits and actions. As your awareness expands, the transformation empowers you on your journey. Learning about your emotions can deepen your awareness of how you feel and this will help you to develop boundaries as you move forward.

One of the most important things a coach will do is to reflect on the things you often say and think that work against you in achieving your goals. As the captain of the ship (your body), the messages you speak internally or externally give directions to your mind. The words used are critical to wellness and abundance.

Saying things like: "I am sick and tired of this," "I will never get ahead," "I am no good" and "I will only screw it up" are all examples of statements that are detrimental to you. These are all common examples of dialogue that send negative "orders" to the mind. Our minds then carry them out and they become self-fulling prophecies. Our mind doesn't know the difference between imagined thought and real experience thought because the brain experiences both real and imagined thoughts in the same way.

A Magnetic Resonance Imaging (MRI) scan is used to show the brain's activity under various conditions. Interestingly the brain lights up in the same brain regions for reality as it does imagination. This means that in a very real way, the brain cannot tell the difference between what is true and what is imagined. Amazing, right?

To further reinforce this idea, studies have shown that athletes who are imagining practicing in their minds show the same successful outcome as athletes who are actually practicing in real life. Top athletes and their coaches know that it is imperative to visualize the positive outcome they desire and that this will enhance performance on the field.

A coach will help you to learn to use the same techniques as these top performers. l help you to change your mindset so that you can learn and install the habits you want to develop.

For centuries, the human body was thought incapable of running a four-minute mile. Roger Banister did this in a race in 1954. Since 1954 nearly 1500 athletes have succeeded in breaking the limits of the four-minute mile. What held them back before wasn't a real limitation of the human body; it was the belief in a limitation.

Just as the runners began to break the four-minute mile as soon as they saw that it was possible; coaches enable people to break through their perceived limitations in all areas of life.

Coaches help clients to slow down and be fully in the present moment. This allows the clients to examine and organize their thoughts. Then, the client can begin to create goals based on their own unique desires, values and goals.

THE COACHING PROCESS

The coaching process includes:

- Reflecting on past positive achievements;
- Examining beliefs and seeing if there is evidence to support negative beliefs;
- Reviewing or reframing possibilities for positive opportunities and
- Allowing for reflection to connect the dots and see the big picture.

Coaches do not tell clients what to do. Instead, they provide space to help the client achieve the goals they choose.

Coaches can assist you in:

- Defining desired outcomes and vision
- Recognizing willingness, confidence and readiness to make changes
- Increasing knowledge of self
- Challenging beliefs

- Designing a plan to learn the skills needed for success
- Learning how to deal with obstacles
- Brainstorming
- Focusing on strengths and resilience
- Defining actions and next steps
- Celebrating outcomes and building on strengths
- Developing desired habits
- Continuing to learn and grow to reach peak development, wellness and excellence that will be sustainable and that can continue

Coaches can help you do this and so much more. Whatever it is that you need to accomplish, remember there is a coach out there who is going to be able to help you get there even faster than you could on your own.

DEALING WITH OBSTACLES AND LIMITATIONS

Your fight or flight response kicks in when stressed, threatened or angry. It is harder to think logically and therefore you're more likely to react. A coach is skilled in helping you get in touch with your feelings and your experiences. Your coach has tools they can use to help you calm down so that you can find solutions that will help you break through your resistance.

Your coach will help you to examine your beliefs and challenge your limitations. Many limitations are learned in childhood when our parents, teachers or other authority figures told us we couldn't do something. Our experience often trains us to believe we have limitations as well.

Here is an interesting example of a learned limitation: baby elephants in captivity are trained to stay in a small area with a peg with a rope fastened into the ground. The baby elephant learns they cannot pull the peg out and this becomes a strong belief. The same elephant, fully grown, could easily pull that peg out of the earth, but is limited by the younger self's belief and limitation. The adult elephant doesn't even try to remove the peg at all and they remain limited by the belief trained into them during their youth.

Just like the elephant, we, as humans, have many limiting beliefs. We may not even be aware that we have these beliefs because they can be so deeply ingrained. A coach will help you to challenge any limiting beliefs you have. They do this by helping you reflect on your beliefs so that you can decide which ones truly work for you and which ones you need to discard. This allows you to create an entirely new, more empowering mindset.

When it comes to your health, a coach can be invaluable. They will show you how you can overhaul your body, mind and emotions. A coach will help you to examine your diet, your exercise routine and your activity level so you can work to find a system that truly nourishes you. A coach will also help you to calm your mind and learn to deal with your emotions more effectively. A trained health coach can guide you in skill development and will help you develop new sustaining habits and actions as your awareness expands about your emotional, physical, mental and spiritual self.

THREE LEVELS OF TRANSFORMATION

There are three levels of transformation that occur as you transform your life.

The First Level of Transformation: Learn Something New

In the first level of transformation—you learn something new. Your learning may take the form of reading a book, listening to a podcast, or taking an online or in person course. Once you learn the information, though, it might be difficult to actually implement the new skill or technique. A coach can help you to do this.

An example from my life is that I had read a book about how to create a schedule and prioritize tasks. I loved the book and thought the ideas were great, but I was finding it hard to develop the habit. I asked my coach for help and they guided me through evaluating tasks, seeing obstacles and setting boundaries. which helped me make changes and establish new habits.

Another example of this was when I was dealing with a conflict in a relationship or at work. I took a training course and read many books and thought I understood the theory, but putting it into practice was another thing entirely. I kept finding myself caught in the emotions of the situation. My coach taught me tools I could use to de-escalate the situation, which helped me to stay calm and communicate my needs effectively.

These are two examples from my own life of times when a coach helped me take the information I learned and incorporate it into my life.

The Second Level of Transformation: Shift in Perspective

In the second level of transformation, you have a shift in perspective. This is when the lesson actually creates a change in your beliefs. A shift in perspective will enable you to move to more empowering beliefs, which will support the person you are becoming. The process of transformation is the process of shifting one perspective after another until you become a better version of yourself.

My first memorable and significant mindset shift was in a class with Miss Brown, a happy young teacher assigned the task of teaching the first remedial reading program in London, where I lived. I was six years old and suffering from depression and anxiety after a family trauma. I was scared, frustrated, disempowered and I felt unhappy at my lack of reading ability.

Miss Brown changed all of that for me. She had an entirely different approach to solving my reading problem. She was caring and enthusiastic and she infused reading with fun. She taught me to imagine that each book was like an adventure we were able to go on. She showed me how books were windows into new worlds. This created a space for me to relax and feel like I could learn to read. She helped me to shift my mindset from the painful, unpleasant and futile task of reading to enjoying reading. I like to think of this young teacher, who made such a difference in my life, as my first coach.

The Third Level of Transformation: Shift Your Identity

This is where all of your hard work pays off.

Shifting your identity is when you step into the new version of yourself that you had once only imagined. When you shift your identity, you have cleared a lot of your past obstacles and created the habits and behaviors that support the new you. You have learned and integrated all the skills you need to sustain the change. Your habits are now permanent and have become part of your lifestyle.

This is when you become the new you.

For me, the process of changing identity was not easy. I hit many obstacles along the way as I worked to shift into who I wanted to be. With the vision of who I wanted to be and my strong purpose, I was able to stay the course and become the person I dreamed of becoming.

FINAL WORDS

Coaching is holistic. It empowers and supports clients in being the best they can be so they can experience shifts that optimize, fulfill and realize their dreams. Globally this is a new era and we are now working towards collective energy, empowering and finding solutions for a sustainable, healthier planet.

Remember, you are here for a reason. You have a passion and purpose inside you, or the ability to create one. Working with coaches to help you along the way, you can develop empowering self-coaching skills.

Everybody can use a coach. Whether you are an athlete, a businessperson, a parent or a student, coaching can help you. Even coaches engage coaches. There are always things to be learned, transformations to be had and higher levels of growth to be achieved.

Coaches are catalysts that open you up so you can move from pain and poverty to wealth, wellness, abundance and unconditional love. They will help you create the life you dream of.

Finding the right coach is very important. Find a coach who you can trust, who maintains confidentiality and who is a trained professional. Don't be afraid to ask for your coach's credentials. A trained coach will provide a professional agreement outlining boundaries and expectations for both parties to follow. The right coach has knowledge and experience in the area of life in which you want to be coached. They are organized and help you track your progress.

Getting to the desired outcome, an experienced teacher or mentor may show you the way, while a coach inspires the mindset shifts you need to achieve the lifestyle, health and wellness you desire. Before you know it, you are creating your reality and evolving in each stage of life as your demands. Coaches encourage you to learn, grow, show gratitude and live your best life.

As for me, I have been through a long journey of transformation. It has been a journey of learning and growth. I had to release a lot of the things I had once believed in order to become the person I am today. I credit all of my amazing coaches for helping me along the way. I couldn't have done it without them. My coaches have been a gift I gave to myself.

Today, my life is totally different. I am a holistic health coach who is trained in a variety of modalities. I have many tools in my toolchest to help my clients to create the life of their dreams. Each day, as I coach my clients, I am thankful that I decided to take this path. I am now living my purpose by helping others to discover their full potential. It is wonderful to share my knowledge and what I have learned.

Please reach out to me if you have any questions or if you want to connect and share your story with me. I would love to hear from you.

With light and love,
Karen

*Our attitude toward life determines
life's attitude towards us.*

~ EARL NIGHTINGALE

ABOUT THE AUTHOR

Karen Stanton is a trained Business Coach, a Divorce Coach and a Holistic Health and Wellness Coach. She has a 10X Wellness coaching certification and is well versed in all aspects of health and fitness. She is trained in NeuroLinguistic Programming (NLP), Hypnosis and Mental Emotional Release.

Inspired by coaches who made a significant difference in her life, she now helps clients worldwide.

Intuition and listening to her body guided her; trusting her emotions and mental, physical and spiritual awareness helped her navigate through bullying, sickness, depression and abuse as a younger woman. Told she would never pass an exam at school or go to college; Karen completed her B.A. major in psychology from the University of Waterloo and is an Ordained Minister. Karen was Director of Finance for non-profit organizations and worked for Business Services for 20 years. Her passion for learning has been her saving grace, empowering and transforming all areas of life.

Today she is healthier than she has ever been, she enjoys exercising and living life to the full with gratitude in Toronto, Canada.

Contact Information:

Karen Stanton.

www.kstantoncoaching.com

info@kstantoncoaching.com

https://www.instagram.com/kstantoncoaching

PART 6

HEALTH AS A
LIFESTYLE

PART 6: HEALTH AS A LIFESTYLE

The very best thing you can do for yourself is to stop making crazy promises to yourself, stop trying to follow every health craze, stop adopting every fad diet and stop being so hard on yourself. So if you stop doing all that, what should you start doing? Well, you can simply start to simply begin to think about what is healthy for your body, right now, at this point of your life.

Approaching health like this will completely and utterly change your life. You begin by loving yourself and your body exactly how it is right now. Yes, right now! Love your body for getting you this far. And then, make the commitment to nourish your body and treat your body in the very best way you can. You learn about yourself and your habits, love your body and then it is easy to make the choices that will make you healthy and happy.

This is the part of the book where we make health a lifestyle. We begin by looking at your body and how you can have a true conscious connection with your body. This is where you get in touch with what you are doing and what your body actually needs. Once you know this, it is easy to design a program that works for you.

Then we move on to health intelligence which will give you more to think about as you examine where you are and where you want to go. Health intelligence is truly about learning how you got here and where you want to go. Once you know that, you can move towards the healthy body, mind and spirit you dream of.

Finally, we end the book with an overview of what living a holistic life looks like. The goal is extraordinary health and wellness and the way to get there is to have the tools you need to get the health you desire. The final chapter will detail a very simple method to actually institute a health lifestyle which you will be able to maintain for a lifetime. This is where it all comes together. You will learn the tools you need and then you can use them to create your version of a holistic, healthy lifestyle.

You are in the homestretch! Let's do it.

**Knowing others is intelligence;
knowing yourself is true wisdom.
Mastering others is strength; mastering
yourself is true power.**

~Lao Tzu

CHAPTER 29

CONSCIOUS BODY CONNECTION

by Freeman Fung

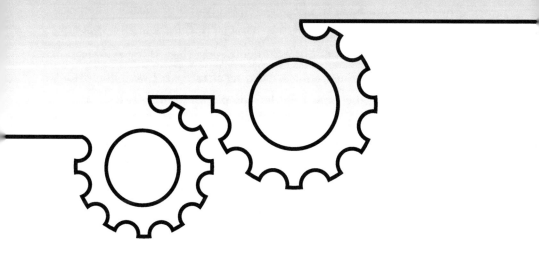

TOPIC:	Holistic Health
TOOL:	Body Mind Connection
TECHNIQUE:	Approach your health from a body, mind and spirit standpoint, understanding that everything in your body is connected.

There are two mistakes along the way to self-mastery:
not starting it and not going all the way.

~ MASTER SHI HENG YI

As a high-achieving globe citizen, I have traveled, backpacked, relocated, lived, studied and worked in over thirty countries and still counting. I am—or was—constantly moving.

For the eight years preceding the closure of international borders due to the COVID-19 were unconsciously built at the expense of my health… back in London in my mid-twenties, I was a business analyst by day and a DJ by night, running at full power—mentally and physically. There was a point where I could have had a long week of deadlines at work, followed by a full-blast Friday night out with my friends, then DJing at a big club the next day and playing until the morning after. After I went home, took a nap, showered and changed, I'd be stomping into the office again, still nailing my Monday presentations.

Then the week continued on. I had so much energy, I wouldn't even feel tired. I had taken more out of alcohol than alcohol had taken out of me!

That's why I always told myself, "I'll rest when I'm dead".

I thought I was at the top of my game—a superhuman who had it all. After all, growing up in Hong Kong and living in this fast-paced 24/7 world, time was the only real currency to me and I couldn't get enough.

All this time, Ironically, this mindset was going to try to get me there much quicker… a series of surprises began to show up after I was transferred to Singapore: I caught myself stopping in the middle of the street—"Where am I going again?" I couldn't remember… or I would be in the grocery store—"What is that one thing I came here to get…?"

At night, I also started developing serious insomnia. "What's wrong with me? Why am I not falling asleep?" Even if I did fall asleep, I kept waking up in the middle of the night, or the next morning I'd wake with agitating thoughts—"What's happening to me? Why am I feeling so fatigued?" From the outside, I had been crowned as a successful, young, high-functioning individual, living a life my peers back home could only dream of. But from the inside, I was silently "disintegrating". Eventually I couldn't physically drag myself out of bed anymore—"Why is my body dragging my life down?"

FROM SURVIVING TO THRIVING

Like most people living in the westernized world, my immediate reaction was to "of course" seek a medical expert. Frustratingly, I only kept getting told by various doctors, all from different countries, that there is no treatment for my Chronic Fatigue Syndrome (CFS). In an attempt to fix my insomnia and serious sleeping problems, I had been taking more than eight different types of sleeping pills and antidepressant drugs, as well as crazy doses of melatonin. Still, none of them helped, but made me feel worse.

As the Chinese proverb goes, "Paper can't wrap up a fire". The final blow eventually came when I was 28, after moving from Singapore to Sydney. I was drained from dealing with the relocation, trying to prove myself at a new job and finding new accommodations within a tight period of time. I also arrived at the time of the Australian bushfires and then went straight into lockdown because of COVID-19. I was shattered. My whole body completely shut down... At that rock bottom, I was shouting for help, desperately. I don't want to live the rest of my life like this! I had no choice but to slow down everything in life, while I was angrily hating my symptoms, my conditions and my body. Only if someone could give me a magical pill to "fix" my health—happily ever after!

Until it finally dawned on me—no one else could really help me if I didn't want to help myself first. That is, I began to realize that I had more responsibility to take care of my body than I had been admitting! I started to accept my past understanding of health might have been flawed—that everything would be okay while I was young, regardless of the extensive alcohols I drank, the late-night partying in clubs and the non-stop traveling...

Why was I always treating the symptoms one by one, but never looking into the root cause? Why couldn't I just prevent the illnesses from happening, rather than finding treatments only after something "goes wrong"? Perhaps my body wasn't the enemy here, but there was something else I was missing? It was through these reflections, I accepted the fact that I also had to make my own efforts to take control of my health.

Thankfully, soon after making this decision, I also learned to develop one of the most transformative techniques for my health and well-being that has turned my life inside out: cultivating a conscious connection with the body. I know, I know—it may sound too simple at first, but yet, it's incredibly powerful. The best of all? It's a free tool! There is no membership to pay, no service to subscribe, but simply an awakening of awareness to bring into your life.

Once you learn to establish this conscious relationship through self-mastery, actions and habits, acquiring extraordinary health also naturally follows.

Not only is my CFS finally gone, I am able to optimize my sleep and have transformed my dreamlife. I have gained so much more energy—physically, mentally and spiritually, rarely have a mood swing and could work less but accomplish way more than that immature "I'll rest when I'm dead" me.

Today, I also have the utmost joy and honor to also transform the well-being of others as a Certified Life Coach with Mindvalley, alongside other holistic authors of this book. Because to me—what good is it to the world if the global citizens living here are always tired, cranky and living in survival mode? Know that it doesn't matter where you are at with your health journey right now, we all have the ability to become a better version of ourselves and thrive in life.

To empower you to build this conscious connection with your own body and to help you to see what is already within you, I have broken this technique down into a simple three-steps process to follow.

BUILDING A CONSCIOUS CONNECTION TO YOUR BODY

Step 1: Be Aware of Your Body's Intelligence

After the first Sydney lockdown, I moved to the Olympic Park and had the opportunity to learn martial arts from Sifu Micke Hoong, who was trained in Singapore under the famed Shaolin Warrior Monk tradition (Direct 49th Generation from the Bodhidharma).

Despite knowing his background, I was still skeptical at first when he told me he managed to recover by himself from more than twenty fractures, slipped discs and joint dislocations throughout his thirty-six years of training. How is that even possible without the help of a surgeon? I kept thinking. But as our training continued through the months, the Shaolin philosophy opened up a new worldview in me.

First of all, Shaolin's teachings on martial arts are not about fighting or winning a championship, but a spiritual practice (that's not necessarily religious) to create a balanced mind, body and spirit. The moves emulate the movements of animals and help us find harmony within ourselves and become one with nature. You see, those unbelievable demonstrations by Shaolin monks on TV, from breaking rocks with their bare hands to bending spears with their skin, are not merely stunts. They are the result of years of extraordinary commitment to practice self-control to be in tune with the body, which eventually looks to us like they're defying physics!

While you and I are likely not planning to train ourselves into a full-time warrior monk, the day-to-day lesson we could definitely take away is: our body is way more intelligent than what we normally give it credit for. If we pause for a second and listen inwards, the fact that our heart is beating and keeping us alive without us needing to worry about it, is a miracle! How ignorant I was to take it for granted that I could breathe, sense, move, digest—not to mention the abilities of detoxifying all the liquor I chucked and regenerating all the neurons I killed! The body is so brilliant. It does a million things without us even thinking about it.

Consider this: When you cut your finger, did you ever need to get into the process of clotting the blood, forming the scab or growing new skin? No! That's the intelligent body at work. Our human body is designed to heal itself. On the other hand, isn't it true that the more you try to poke the wound and intervene the healing, the longer it takes for it to repair? What I realized is that the same goes with my symptoms I was hating—the chronic fatigue, brain fog or insomnia, were all my own doing that kicked my body out of balance cumulatively throughout the years, without me being aware of it. I was unintentionally blind! That is all to say, consciously recognising there is an innate intelligence inside us is the essential first step for holistic healing.

Here, I want to stretch your mind even further. Did you know your skin sheds approximately 40,000 cells every minute (that is 50 million cells per day!) and replaces them with healthy cells? If you lay out the blood vessels in your body side by side, the string would be long enough to wrap around the Earth 2.5 times (~100,000km)? If a neuron is stimulated through electrical impulses, your brain's information could travel up to an impressive 268 miles per hour?

American stem cell biologist and epigenetics pioneer, Dr. Bruce Lipton, once pointed out, "If you look at yourself in the mirror and see yourself as a single entity, it's a total misperception. The simple truth is you're made out of 50 trillion cells. The cells are the living entity. You, by absolute definition, are a community." So by this perspective, as you say my name, "Freeman," you're not really addressing me as a single entity. You're addressing a community of 50 trillion intelligent citizens! And there are not just human cells—approximately two pounds of our body mass is from a microbiome: the community of bacteria, viruses and fungi that perform a variety of functions for our body, which are all part of the complex ecosystem we cannot live without!

These are more than scientific fun facts I am sharing with you. Your body temple is so much more than just the meat. There are intricate, beautiful and powerful mechanisms with natural orders behind all these, where even science cannot explain yet. Let's not take it for granted. And now that you acquired this expanded awareness of your body's intelligence, it's time to build this trust further.

Step 2: Become Your Body's Best Friend

Just imagine for a second, what would you want your ideal friend to be like? Would you like them always bringing you out to try the best food in town? Always available for you when you need something? Your time together is filled with only joy and laughter? Support you with compassion and kindness whenever you are feeling down?

Most people would instantly say yes to all these questions. But interestingly, when we flip it around and consider your body as "the friend" here instead, how often do we treat it in the same manner? Well, the answers are pretty obvious (and unfortunate) when we look at the alarming statistics on lifestyle diseases: According to the World Health Organization (WHO), cardiovascular diseases are the leading cause of death globally, taking an estimated 17.9 million lives each year, most of which can be prevented. While back in 1980, the world had around 108 million cases of diabetes—in 2019, an estimated 1.5 million deaths were directly caused by diabetes across the globe.

The statistics on the struggles people have with sleep are staggering. Insomnia affects between 30% to 45% of our adult population nowadays and it's been reported that roughly 62% of adults worldwide feel that they don't sleep well when they go to bed…But not you—not after reading this chapter and making the mindset shift to see your body as your friend and to take care of it well.

Next time when you feel tempted to stay up late watching "one more" episode of your favorite show, I encourage you to ask: Can I actually watch this tomorrow and let my best friend take some rejuvenating rest first? And even if you decided to make changes but then backslide for whatever reason, can I encourage you not to beat yourself up—and thank your body with compassion and self-love? Living in this 24/7 non-stop culture, too many people push and push themselves to the point of exhaustion, as if they'll win some sort of award for trying the hardest.

People who sleep less are praised for being tough. People don't mind putting poison into their bodies day-to-day, but they blame the medical system when things go south. I get it. I really do—I have been there myself too and spent enough painful years in this stupid self-inflicted war. But we all have the potential to transform. Be conscious that your body is not your enemy but your best friend—your body intelligence will also react in a positive way to self-heal and self-renew.

Step 3: Cultivate a Deep and Long-term Relationship

Most people (including my old self) just want a quick fix to their problems. But the truth is, cultivating health and wellness requires self-knowledge, self-experimentation, self-reflection and time. Like any other healthy relationship, it does take continuous efforts to nurture. But worry not, the journey could be filled with fun too! Looking back on my health path—fascinatingly enough, I never expected learning martial arts was just a one small first step I took. As soon as I consciously started taking full responsibility for my well-being, there was no stopping a human mind.

The next thing I knew, instead of ordering takeaways and eating my favorite pasta three times a day, I found myself cooking and preparing meals. I become curious to read more and more about what high performers do with their diets and health routines. Gradually, my commitment to health led me to begin a biohacking journey.

Biohacking is the process of using science and technology to better understand and self-improve one's own biology. That could be from making lifestyle changes, listening to functional audio to boost performance, to using wearable tech to track your biometrics.

In a sense, we are consciously improving our relationship with the body through bringing in constant upgrades.

Excitingly, knowledge itself is now global—that is, the sum total of human knowledge is available to us. We have access to information—from ancient to modern, East to West—way beyond what schools, societies or news covered. So with a world of information available at our fingertips (and thanks to the work of pioneer biohackers such as Dave Asprey, the founder of the Bulletproof brand and Upgrade Labs), we literally have access to more health and nutritional information than any of the presidents in the world twenty years ago!

Starting with one small step at a time, today my health has changed in ways I never thought possible. I enjoy a clean and, whenever possible, organic diet (or lifestyle, I should say)—processed food free, artificial junk free, sugar free, unhealthy fats free, industrial meat free, gluten free—which couples with intermittent fasting. I wear bluelight-blocking glasses after sundown to protect my natural melatonin secretions, alongside a wind-down hour before bed that includes meditation, red light therapy and journaling a gratitude list. I bought myself a wearable sleep tracker as well, so I could quantify my sleep data by measuring metrics like sleep efficiency, sleep stages and HRV (Heart Rate Variability).

Besides adopting these "universal biohacks", I also did tests such as DNA sequencing, IgG food sensitivity, heavy metal testing and microbiome mapping to understand my individual biology. I practice breathwork (like the Wim Hof Method) together with cold therapy to combat my seasonal sinusitis and allergies instead of abusing antibiotics. I invest in a cupboard full of supplements, all at my disposal to boost my immune system, gut health and training recovery—or to simply minimize my risk from bad food when dining out. Because really, there is no contradiction between living a healthy life and socializing with friends once you learn how to optimize and be in tune with your body. We can find the balance in all things.

To be very clear, I'm not asking you to blindly follow my health regime and I'm not saying you should ignore what your medical advisor tells you. But I am encouraging you to start cultivating a better connection with your body. Study your own biology, experiment with what works best for your individual health and cater to your own optimisation goals and needs, for the longer term. I know this could be a lot to absorb, but the bottom line is—not only do you have the power to help prevent illness from manifesting in your body, but you also have the power to promote your vitality and life span!

In fact, what I shared here is just a sliver of what one could adopt in the world of biohacking, let alone to mention the exponential speed of technological development happening as you are reading this. Isn't that exhilarating—there are limitless potentials waiting to upgrade our body and cultivate the ultimate well-being?

And after understanding the basis of these three steps, from my coaching experiences, chances are—there was at least one thing already popped up in your head—that one thing you always knew is good for your health and you wanted to try, but always managed to find an excuse not to. What is it? Could this be your next precious gift you give to yourself?

YOUR TURN TO THRIVE

Is health and well-being an area of life you're carefully cultivating, or something you tend to "fix" only after something goes wrong? How would it feel if you could live your life with radiant health—feeling strong, energized and vibrant?

It's time to question this time-famine culture, unplug ourselves from obsolete routines and stop distracting ourselves with constant motion. It's time to take control of our bodies through self-mastery. It's time to move to the new paradigm—to focus on creating our wellness and not just treating the illness. Make the lifestyle shift to total well-being. Don't wait for that life-threatening wake-up call. I didn't understand it back then, but now I feel truly grateful. I am truly grateful that I had to experience all those struggles, battles, pain and sleepless nights, so that I could learn, upgrade and transform into who I am today, as well as being able to inspire others to do the same.

Remember, it's not normal to feel tired all the time, regardless of how our on-the-go culture has made it the norm. Spending time on self-care doesn't suggest you are a lazy, unsuccessful, or worthless individual, despite our cultural messages otherwise. You too have the power to turn your body into a high-performance vehicle—work less, achieve more and thrive in this modern world.

I look forward to meeting the best version of yourself out in the world one day!

WIth love,
Freeman

The greatest crime in the world is to not develop your potential. When you do what you do best, you are helping not only yourself, but the world.

~ROGER WILLIAMS

ABOUT THE AUTHOR

Freeman Fung is an international author, speaker and certified life coach who has advocated new global citizenship at TEDx, Mindvalley, world tourism forums and more.

Originally from Hong Kong, he left home solo at age 19 to live in Romania for a Global Village project. He subsequently embarked on a journey to travel and experience life in more than 30 countries (and still counting). While enjoying exploring the world, he is also a passionate photographer, DJ/musician, Shaolin martial artist, biohacker, Mindvalley Ambassador, Integral thinker and lucid dreamer.

A true believer in the power of the mind, with a heart inspired by cultural diversity and inclusion, Freeman is on a mission to awaken more world citizens, raise our global consciousness and make the world a better place through personal transformations.

Contact Information:

Website: traveltotransform.com http://traveltotransform.com/

LinkedIn:https://www.linkedin.com/in/freeman-fung/

**Power will accomplish much,
but perseverance more.**

~William Scott Downey

No one is born fully-formed: it is
through self-experience in the world
that we become what we are.

~Paulo Freire

CHAPTER 30
HEALTH INTELLIGENCE

by Irma Nejstgaard

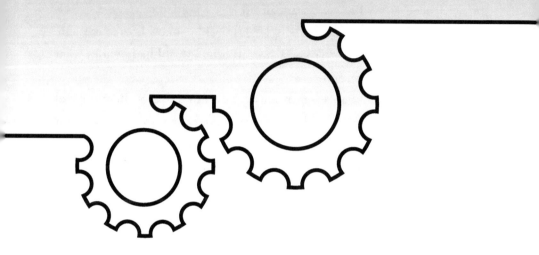

TOPIC:	Holistic Intelligence
TOOL:	Awareness, Knowledge, Self Care
TECHNIQUE:	Learn the basics of health and wellness in order to implement the self care methods that work for you.

Nothing is particularly hard if you divide it into small jobs.

~ HENRY FORD

My health journey started in earnest a few years after I moved to Denmark. I had taken a conscious parenting course, which made me realize that my behavior, beliefs and patterns of living would be passed on to my children. It made me think about what I wanted for my kids and I realized that above all, I wanted them to be healthy and happy. This meant that they needed to have a healthy body and a healthy mind.

I looked at my lifestyle and realized that I needed to change. I realized that I didn't know much about health. I didn't know how to measure health and I certainly didn't know how healthy I was. I had no idea what healthy living really meant.

I was healthier than I had been in my younger years. Before I had moved to Denmark I was working too many hours, many of them at night and my schedule was often thrown off. I would periodically try different diets and exercise routines, but nothing lasted. I was smoking at that time and completely ignoring my health. I was stressed and I found myself sinking into depression at one point.

I remember one of my patients during that time was a very wealthy Danish man. He was in his mid-eighties at the time I worked for him. Although he was incredibly wealthy, he was not happy. He was lonely and sick.

One day I asked him if he was happy he had accumulated that much money. He didn't answer at first, but then a very sad look came over his face. He said, "There was no purpose to accumulating all this money. No reason at all." That stuck with me. I realized then that it wasn't money that could make you healthy or happy. I think that is when I began to think I should take better care of myself.

That was when I started learning about health. I found out that six out of ten deaths among Europeans aged 70-90 are due to the fact that the individuals did not practice a healthy lifestyle. I learned that lifestyle and environment accounted for 90-95% of our most chronic illnesses according to the National Library of Medicine.

Isn't that crazy?

I wanted to keep learning so I dove right in. I wanted to become healthier for myself and for my children. I wanted to be a good role model and in order to do that, I needed to be educated.

In 2020 I enrolled in a health school in Denmark. At the same time I invested in holistic health-longevity and science-based courses and I loved what I was learning. I completed my education by reading books about physical and mental health.

No matter how much I learned, I wanted to know more. I felt I was hungry for knowledge because now I wanted to implement a healthier lifestyle. I kept learning and growing and it was a great feeling. I finally started to have a clear vision for what living a healthy lifestyle looked like. I was ready to implement it in my life.

WHY WE LIVE UNHEALTHY LIFESTYLES

We live in a time where there is a plethora of information about healthy living. We have all the information we could ever want at our fingertips. The resources are endless online and all we need to do is look for it.

So why do we continue to propagate unhealthy lifestyles?

There are a few reasons for that.

The first reason is that we are all raised with a system of beliefs about health and wellness. We learn these from our families, from our friends and from the society around us. Additionally, we have plenty of companies that are selling us products that are not good for us. Add to this all the competing information about what is and what is not healthy and you can see why it is difficult to find a healthier way of living.

The second reason is that we tend to stick with what we know because it is comfortable. We continue on with the same habits that got us into the health situation we are currently in because that is what we know. It is often easier to stick with what you know than what you don't know. Thus, we resist change because change is uncomfortable.

The third reason is that moving from an unhealthy to a healthy life-style takes a lot of learning, commitment and motivation. It seems like a huge mountain to climb, so we choose to stay where we are.

HEALTHY LIFESTYLE CHOICES

So how do we do it? How do we make healthier lifestyle choices? We must begin with awareness, knowledge and self care.

AWARENESS

In order to live a long and healthy life in our society, we need to raise our awareness around our health. This is the first step and it takes the desire to be honest with yourself about where you are.

In this stage, you examine your physical health by looking at your weight, the shape of your body and how your body feels. You determine how much muscle you have and how much fat you have. You might want to do a test like a DEXA scan, where they determine where the fat on your body is distributed and how much muscle mass you have. This is crucial information for you and will give you a nice baseline to start.

During this stage of awareness, you look at your nutrition first. You want to determine if your diet consists of mostly processed foods or mostly whole foods. An easy way to do this is to look at the food you currently have in your house. Processed foods are foods that come in boxes, cans or bags and they have long lists of ingredients. Whole foods are foods close to their natural form with very few ingredients. Ideally, you want to eat less processed foods and more natural foods.

Hydration is super important too. Are you drinking lots of sugary drinks or drinks with a lot of caffeine? For optimal health, you want to drink mostly water so that you can hydrate your body properly.

Look at your level of activity next. Are you active or mostly passive? Do you exercise regularly? Are you doing both strength training and cardiovascular training? Do you spend time outdoors doing fun, active hobbies and sports?

Be kind to yourself as you develop a true awareness of your current state of health. Remember to be proud of yourself that you are beginning to take responsibility for your health. Keep a positive attitude no matter where you are.

Cultivating Awareness

1. Physical Health
   a. Do a full body assessment by measuring and noting:
      i. Your weight
      ii. Your body size and shape
         1. Take photos of your body from the front, the back and each side.
         2. Take photos of your face from the front and each side.
         3. These photos will serve as the before pictures, a baseline for where you are beginning.
      iii. Your body mass index (BMI)
         1. Although this measurement is not one of the more accurate ways to gauge overall health, it is a good indicator if you do not have access to a dexa scan.
      iv. Body Fat
         1. Calipers can give a rough estimate of your body fat percentage
         2. DEXA scan: this is a great way to get an amazing view of the distribution of your fat throughout your body. You will receive a body scan and a full printout showing you exactly where your fat deposits are.
            a. A key health indicator is the level of fat in your abdominal area and around your organs.
            b. A DEXA scan will show you exactly how much fat is in your abdominal area.

v. General Level of Fitness
   1. How is your cardiovascular health?
      a. A visit to the cardiologist will give you a great overview of this area of your health, as well as providing a baseline measurement.
   2. What is your overall level of muscle distribution throughout your body?
2. Mental Health
   a. What is your level of mental health?
   b. Do you experience mostly positive emotions or mostly negative emotions?
   c. Are you able to function and fulfill your obligations each day?

Knowledge

Once you have become aware of your health status, it is time to gain the knowledge you need to create the healthy state you desire.

Luckily, we live in a day and age where all the knowledge you need is right there on your phone or computer. You can begin by searching the internet for information on nutrition, hydration and exercise. Look for videos, podcasts, blogs, articles and online courses on the topic you want to learn about. Buy books about health to expand your knowledge.

Make sure that you incorporate the things you are learning into your life. Start by making one small change and let that become a part of your life before you make the next change. Go easy on yourself since you are at the beginning of your health transformation. It is best to have consistency with small changes and to make those habits before you attempt to make bigger changes.

Make sure that you celebrate each new habit you install. Congratulate yourself and share your wins with the people around you. Keeping a positive attitude by celebrating your wins will create a lot of motivation to continue on your journey.

Increasing Your Knowledge

Educate yourself on the areas of health that you want to work on. If you are interested in improving your nutrition, you can learn anything you need to know by going online and watching podcasts, masterclasses and videos. You can read articles and books on nutrition as well.

As you study nutrition, focus on finding an eating plan that works for you and works for your body. Remember, each person is different, so it is imperative that you find the foods that work for you. Make sure that the plan you pick works for your lifestyle so that it will be sustainable.

When you are ready to learn about the fitness aspect of your health, keep in mind that you want to find an exercise that works for you. Watch a few different exercise videos and see what type of exercise might interest you. You want to find an exercise routine that you find fun so that you will be able to maintain the program. There are countless types of exercise that you can bring into your life.

The main thing you want to do is to begin. Once you have learned what you need to know, implement the exercise routine into your life. Do that routine for a few weeks in order to see if it is something you want to continue. Remember to start slow, especially if you are starting an exercise routine for the very first time.

Selfcare

Your body is the only place you live. So it is essential to take care of it.

Ask yourself these questions first:

1. What is my relationship with my body?
2. How do I treat my body?
3. Do I appreciate my body?

Do some journaling to understand how you really feel about your body. Be honest as you journal so that you can get a clear view of how you think about your body. Once you have done this, you are ready to practice self care.

Self Care Practices:

- Journaling
- Meditation
- Stretching, Yoga or Qi Gong
- Taking a bath
- Getting a massage
- Taking a walk
- Listening to music
- Dancing
- Spending time in nature
- Nurturing your relationships
- Creating an oasis of peace and calm in your bedroom
  - Declutter
  - Put up room darkening shades
  - Add candles, beautiful lighting and incense
  - Buy new sheets, blanket and pillows

These are just a few ideas for self care. Keep in mind that self care encompasses anything that nourishes and replenishes you. Experiment until you find your own self care practices that help you feel great! I would love to hear from you, please reach out to share your feedback and your journey.

All my love,
Irma

Believe in your heart that you're meant to live a life
full of passion, purpose, magic and miracles.

~ ROY T. BENNETT

ABOUT THE AUTHOR

Irma grew up in Klaipeda, Lithuania. She moved to Denmark in 2012, where she worked in nursing homes. This led her to enroll in health school where she learned about all aspects of health and wellness. She has completed many health courses and holds certifications in health care and holistic coaching.

Irma now works as a holistic health coach and a longevity fitness coach. Her three core values are: awareness, creativity and love.She uses her extensive knowledge to guide people towards their healthiest selves.

Contact Information:
Website: https://holocoach.webnode.dk/
Email: holocoachdk@gmail.com
Instagram: @irmanejstgaard

Envision the grandest vision for the greatest
version of your most vibrant health.
Hold this vision in your mind until it is a
glimmering, shimmering image.
Allow this image to guide you as you
prepare and eat your meals.
Let it guide you in your pursuit
of exercise and activity.
Hold strong to this vision for
every decision you make
and you will one day wake up and find
yourself living health as a lifestyle.
And that, my friends, is when life becomes magical.

~Kerry Fisher

CHAPTER 31

TOOLS FOR EXTRAORDINARY LIVING

by Kerry Fisher

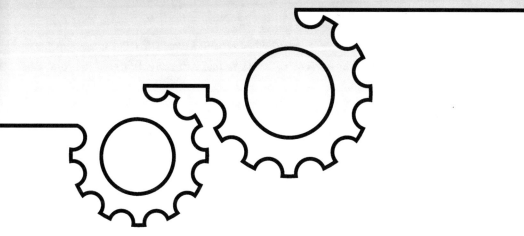

TOPIC:	Healthy Lifestyle
TOOL:	Holistic Wellness
TECHNIQUE:	Weaving health and wellness into your life so that it is no longer a practice, it is a lifestyle.

Living a holistic lifestyle means that you are taking care of your body, mind and spirit. Embracing vibrant health becomes a part of the fabric of your life.

~KERRY FISHER

I was a competitive gymnast throughout my childhood. I was lucky because I had a fantastic coach who influenced my entire life.

My coach, Diane, was a force of nature. She was a former competitive gymnast and her love of gymnastics had inspired her to open a gym in my town. I spent most of my childhood there in that gym and it is where I learned the most important life lessons I needed to learn.

Diane was a badass. She was a tall, willowy blonde with a muscular, athletic body. She could run in heels and she taught us how to do that too. She was my hero. There was nothing she couldn't do. One time I asked her how she was so good at everything and she looked at me and said just one word, "Practice."

She was a dedicated coach who taught us all the techniques we needed to learn to be great technical gymnasts. Beyond that, she taught us how to love our bodies and how to take care of them. She taught us everything we needed to know about health and wellness and I owe her a debt of gratitude for that.

Diane was a woman ahead of her time. She had an innate grasp of how the body worked. She taught us that everything was connected. She explained that our body and mind worked together to create our physical and mental state. Diane taught us about mindset and how to visualize as well as how we had to think about nutrition and exercise as a way to keep our body healthy. It was a unique perspective, especially back then, because she didn't focus on calories or on weight. Instead, she focused on health.

I grew up wanting to take care of my body. I made sure that I ate healthy foods, drank lots of water and that I was active every day. I also focused on dealing with my emotions by paying attention to how I was feeling. I have never gone on a diet or deprived myself of anything. I haven't spent hours and hours in the gym working out and trying to be healthy. Instead, I have focused on living a healthy lifestyle throughout my days, weeks, months and years.

Today I am 55 years old. I am the mother of five and I have a career I absolutely love. I am in great health and in shape and I have the same energy levels I did as a young woman. I am sure that this is because of all those lessons

I learned in the gym all those years ago from my beautiful coach Diane. I am grateful that I learned to take care of myself from such a young age, which is why I am motivated to teach this style of living to others.

HOLISTIC LIFESTYLE

Living a healthy lifestyle should be a joyous journey.
~ KERRY FISHER

What is a holistic lifestyle? A holistic lifestyle is one where you have vibrant physical, emotional, mental and spiritual health. Your physical body is strong, you have a balanced diet, you stay hydrated and you have a healthy exercise routine. Your mental and emotional health is strong as well. You know how to handle your emotions, even when life gets tough. You have stress relief practices that you use when you need them. Your spiritual health is good too. Spiritual health is when you feel at ease, in flow and connected to the world around you.

I know, I know, it seems impossible to live a life like that. How can you possibly live a life of equanimity where you float through the ups and downs of life? Is it even possible to attain a lifestyle like this? It is possible, but it does take work.

I want to take a moment here to say that this does not mean that life will be all butterflies and roses. We all have obstacles we will bump up against, difficulties that will arise and people that will challenge us. This is life. It is natural to have ups and downs. We are human. We can't avoid this.

What I am saying, though, is that you can learn to live a life where health and wellness is woven into the fabric of your life. A life where you don't have to worry about your weight or health because you eat a diet that nourishes you. A life where your body is strong because you are active and exercise is a part of your everyday routine. A life where you can handle whatever comes your way because you have the emotional strength and the tools you need to deal with those inevitable challenges.

This is what I mean by living a holistic lifestyle. It's not living a life where everything is perfect. It's living a life that no matter what happens, you are still healthy and happy.

Are you ready to weave wellness into your life? Let's do it!

TOOLS FOR EXTRAORDINARY LIVING

I couldn't resist titling this chapter *Tools for Extraordinary Living* because this is the way I seek to live. It is also what I teach, write about and speak about. I specialize in teaching people simple tools for bringing wellness practices into their life. I like to emphasize the word simple because everything I teach is a tool that is easy to incorporate into your life. I believe healthy living should be fun.

In order to live a healthy lifestyle, you must create healthy habits that support you. The pillars of a great lifestyle include having a morning routine and an evening routine; making sure you pay attention to your nutrition and hydration; having stress reduction techniques that you can use when you feel overwhelmed; improving your relationships; and creating a beautiful home. Once those things are in place, you can focus on improving your quality of life and developing a life vision so that you are living a life of purpose.

This is the basic overview for living a holistic lifestyle. It may seem a bit overwhelming to see that list but have no fear, I will give you a brief overview of each topic and some simple tools so that you can begin to add these healthy habits into your life slowly over time. Remember, small changes over time have huge results.

MORNING ROUTINE

Imagine if you could start every day with peace and ease. Well, you can, using a simple technique called *The Snooze Button Technique*. I created the *Snooze Button Technique* years ago as a way to help my clients take action and begin to actually add wellness practices into their life.

So what is the *Snooze Button Technique?* Well, it's simple. When your alarm goes off in the morning, you simply reach over, hit the snooze button, but instead of going back to sleep you get up and do something that makes you feel good. You can exercise or stretch, do yoga or Qi Gong, meditate or do breathwork, dance or listen to music, journal or just stare out the window. It doesn't really matter what you choose to do in the morning, What matters is that you get up and you do it.

I have taught this technique to my clients, friends and family for years. It works!

The reason it works is that we are utilizing something we all do which is hit the snooze button and use it as a trigger to do something that nurtures us. It is easy to remember and easy to do. It's great because you begin your day with a win. You have already done something to take care of yourself and this creates a wonderful feeling for you to start your day with.

It's a lot better than hitting the snooze button ten times, finally getting up, realizing you are running late and then racing around trying to get yourself up and out.

The Snooze Button Technique is a great way to begin a morning routine. Try it.

EVENING ROUTINE

Creating an evening routine is just as important as creating a morning routine.

In order to create a great evening routine, begin by designating a period of time before bed that you are willing to designate as your evening routine time. It is wise to start with a short time period like 15 minutes and once you have mastered that, increase the time until you have a nice solid one hour routine before bed.

So what do you do during your evening routine?

Break this time into three sections.

The first part is your preparation for the following day. Take out your clothes for the morning as well as getting your briefcase, car keys and anything else you may need in the morning ready. You might want to set up the coffee machine or set the table for breakfast. Prepare your house for slumber by turning off the overhead lights and transitioning into a nice, relaxing lighting state.

The next part of your evening routine is focused on hygiene. This is when you brush your teeth, wash your face and take care of your physical body. You might shower or take a bath during this period. You can take the time to use lotion or a delicious body oil and massage your feet to really feel great.

Finally, the third section of time is your relaxation time. You can read a book, journal or listen to music during this time. This might be time to reconnect with your lover, taking a few minutes to spend time together. You could stretch or do some light yoga. You might want to take a moment to think about what you are grateful for, or to think about what went right during the day. Moving into a positive mindset prior to sleep is a fabulous way to ensure a great night's rest.

Those are the elements of an evening routine, but don't feel like you have to limit yourself to these suggestions. Create an evening routine that works for you, one that will help you end the day in the same lovely way you began it. With peace and calm.

Once you have installed morning and evening routines, you will begin and end your days in a fantastic way. You might not be able to control what happens when you leave your house during the day, but you sure can control what happens at the beginning and end of your day. Make these times work for you.

NUTRITION AND HYDRATION

There is endless advice on nutrition and hydration that you can follow. It is important for you to learn about these topics so that you can figure out what works for you.

My best advice in the area of health and nutrition is for you to remember that you only have one body so you might as well take care of it. Approaching nutrition and hydration as a way to take care of your body will help you make healthy choices throughout the day. Instead of focusing on numbers or calories, focus on health. Anytime you eat or drink something, ask yourself if this is something that will nourish your body. This is a gentle way to think about food.

The simplest nutrition advice of all is to eat nutritious, whole foods. This means eating foods that are as close to their natural state as possible. Fruits, vegetables and proteins are all whole foods. Avoid processed foods as much as possible. It might seem like these foods are easier to prepare, but it is helpful to ask yourself if the long term health effects of the processed foods are worth the ease of preparation. Think about what will happen to your body if you keep eating those boxed, canned and pre-prepared foods. Is it really worth it?

In order to make it simple, try to cook in bulk. Every few days, cook in batches. On these preparation days, you can cut vegetables and prepare foods that are healthy. This makes it easier to maintain a healthy diet.

Finally, drink plenty of water. If you currently drink lots of sugary drinks, begin by replacing one of these and once you have done that, wait a few days and replace the next sugary drink. Slowly, over time, switch to drinking mostly water.

STRESS REDUCTION TECHNIQUES

Find stress reduction tools that work for you. Meditation and breathwork are two simple, easy to learn techniques that you can introduce into your life. For an easy meditation, simply close your eyes and concentrate on the breath coming in and out of your nose. Focus only on the breath and when you find your attention drifting off, bring your attention gently back to the breath. This is a simple, easy to use meditation that will make you feel great. You can do it for a minute or more. Try it and see how you feel after you practice. You can also find meditation apps and guided meditation videos online.

Breathwork is another great stress reduction tool. Try the box breath technique, which was created by the NAVY Seals. Box breathing is easy. Breathe in for a count of 4, hold your breath for a count of 4, breath out for a count of 4 and then hold your breath out for a count of 4. That is one round. Repeat 3-5 rounds and notice the effect.

There are plenty of other stress reduction tools you can use. It might be journaling or practicing gratitude. Maybe calling a friend or checking in with a relative will lift your spirits. You can take a walk or sit and watch the sunset. Find what works for you.

RELATIONSHIPS

Examining your relationships is a key part of health that we often overlook. It is said that you are the sum total of the five people you spend the most time with, but I would say that you are the sum total of *all* the people you spend time with. Ultimately, we are affected by the people we work with, live with and spend our leisure hours with. Our family, friends, neighbors and coworkers all affect our state of mind. And our state of mind affects our physical health.

This might seem harsh, but it is essential to examine your relationships. Think about everyone in your life and think about whether spending time with these people makes you feel good or makes you feel bad. Be honest. Spend more time with the people that uplift you and less with the people that drag you down.

Doing a relationship audit like this might be the gamechanger you need to create a completely different life. Be brave and try it.

YOUR CAREER

Do you love your career? Do you hop out of bed every day, eager to get to work? Eager to work your craft? If you do, congratulations! If you don't love your career, then it is time to find a side passion, a passion project.

What is a passion project? Well, a passion project is a side project which inspires and motivates you. A side project where you are doing something that you absolutely love doing. This is where you can use the skills that you don't get to use at work, so that you can create something that makes you feel fulfilled.

A side project is a nice way to begin to work on things you are interested in but that you are not sure you can make enough money to support yourself with. You can dedicate a few hours a week to working on your side project and build it slowly. The nice thing about a side project is that it allows you to work on a new project without all the pressure to make money, or make the side project a success.

Have you always wanted to be a speaker or a writer? Perhaps you have dreamed of becoming a yoga teacher or fitness instructor. Or maybe you want to become a coach. Or an artist, jewelry maker or a pottery maker. The possibilities are endless.

To start, make a list of everything you are interested in. Don't limit yourself, simply allow the ideas to flow. Then, look at the list and see if there are any common threads. See if any of the things on the list really leap out at you and make you excited. Then, try it and see if you like it, if it sparks your passion. If it does, keep going, if not, try something new.

Allow yourself the luxury of experimenting as you look for a passion project. Don't put any pressure on yourself. Once you find something that really sparks your interest, take classes and learn as much as you can about it. Then practice.

Who knows what could happen!

Your passion project might just become a new career path. You never know.

YOUR HOME

Home sweet home! Make your home your sanctuary. When you enter your home, you want it to feel like a warm hug.

In order to create a home like this, the first step is decluttering. Do yourself a favor and take out all the clutter in your house. Get a laundry basket or a bag and go around, room by room and take out every piece of clutter you see. Check the corners, under the furniture, on every surface and in every drawer. Get it out and sort it in another room. Discard anything you don't need.

As you declutter, give yourself the permission to get rid of anything that doesn't add value to your life. A great book to help you with this process is *The Life-Changing Magic of Tidying Up* by Marie Kondo. She has a fantastic system of decluttering that will have your home clear and organized in no time.

Once you have decluttered, it is time to make your home comfortable and beautiful. Surround yourself with the things that you love. Add small touches like comfortable blankets, throw pillows, candles and scents that will make your home inviting and welcoming.

Your home is your place to recharge and reconnect with yourself. Make it a place of peace and calm, an oasis that perfectly suits you and your family.

QUALITY OF LIFE

Quality of life? Another area that is easy to overlook, but one that is essential to peak health.

Quality of life is having a life filled with adventures, fun and excitement. This is different for each one of us.

For some, a great quality of life means traveling around the world and experiencing new places. For others, a great quality of life is having a gorgeous home and all the toys they could imagine, like a nice car or boat. Still, others might want a vacation home where they can retreat whenever they want.

Whatever your definition of a great quality life is, make a plan so that you can achieve the quality of life you want. Life is meant to be lived, so don't neglect this crucial aspect of ultimate wellness.

LIFE VISION

Life vision is the jewel of the crown of life.

Life vision means having a vision for your life. As you think about your life vision, ask yourself where you want to be in a year, in five years, in ten years and at the end of your life. Imagine looking back on the last day of your life and reflecting on your life, what would you want your life to have looked like?

Life vision encompasses all the categories we talked about earlier in this chapter. It is your health, your relationships, your career, your quality of life. Life vision is the whole package.

Give yourself a few minutes to sit down and write all of the things you want to accomplish, all of the adventures you want to have, all of the aspects of your life that you want to experience during your lifetime. Allow yourself to dream big. Make the grandest vision for the greatest life you can imagine.

As part of creating your grand vision, make sure that you think about your purpose, your mission here on earth. What do you want to give to the world, how do you want to serve? What do you want your life to have stood for? This, my friends, is the key to it all.

Life vision provides the fuel to give us the motivation and the determination to create that life we dream of.

To learn more about the ideas in this chapter, please look for my book, *Routines for Extraordinary Living*. The book will help to create routines that will support you as you move towards creating your most extraordinary life.

FINAL WORDS

You deserve to live the very best life. Did you hear that? Let me say it again, I really want you to take this in. You deserve to live the very best life you can imagine. You do. Yes, you do.

It's up to you, though. You have to make the choice. Nobody can do it for you. Only you can choose to live a life of passion and purpose. Only you can decide that you will have vibrant health all the days of your life. Only you can take the steps you need to create that amazing quality of life and life vision that you want for yourself.

Living a holistic lifestyle is a fantastic way to move towards the very best version of yourself, so that you can create the life of your dreams.

I know that you can do it. And when you do, I would love to hear about it. I would love for you to reach out and tell me your story of success. I want to hear all about how you created the life you dreamed of. And when you do, I shall celebrate with you.

I wish you health, happiness and most of all, I wish you an extraordinary life!

With extraordinary love,
Kerry

You can become the very best version of yourself.
You can live your most extraordinary life.
You can. It's all up to you.

~ KERRY FISHER

ABOUT THE AUTHOR

Kerry is an author, a speaker and a wellness educator. She is a licensed attorney who left her law career to pursue an extraordinary life.

Her mission is to help others find a more balanced and fulfilled life. She believes in action and she teaches Simple Tips for Extraordinary Living using stress reduction techniques and work-life balance to help people supercharge their lives. She coaches corporate clients and elite athletes in mindset and peak performance techniques and creates tailored programs for private clients who are seeking mastery in all areas of their lives.

After many years of teaching and coaching, Kerry is focused on writing, creating courses and speaking on the topics she is so passionate about. She is on a mission to inspire and encourage people to become the person they dream of being and to create the life they imagine.

Contact Information:
Website: kerryfishercoaching.com
Instagram:@kerryfisher
Email: iamkerryfisher@gmail.com
LinkedIn: www.linkedin.com/in/kerry-fisher-

CONCLUSION

Many of life's failures are people who did not realize how close they were to success when they gave up.

~THOMAS A. EDISON

You have done it! You have made it to the end of the book. That shows your motivation and commitment to living a healthy, holistic lifestyle.

No matter what your current health status is today, remember that it is never too late to embrace a holistic lifestyle. It is our hope that the stories in this book have inspired you and motivated you to begin your own health journey. Try the different tips and techniques from this book to create your own perfect health routine.

Be patient with yourself as you begin this new way of living. There will be setbacks, there will be obstacles, there will be times when you feel like giving up. When that happens, remember the stories you read in this book. Let these stories remind you that it is possible to overcome anything. If we can do it, you can do it too.

We honor you and look forward to hearing your amazing stories of transformation. Remember...

You are extraordinary.

With love, light and laughter,
Kerry and Lawrence

Your time is limited, so don't waste it living someone else's life. Don't be trapped by dogma—which is living with the results of other people's thinking.

~Steve Jobs

The following pages contain the introduction to the book *Tools for Extraordinary Living: The Snooze Button Sessions.*

This is the first book in the *Extraordinary Living Trilogy.*

You can find *Tools for Extraordinary Living: The Snooze Button Sessions* and the second book in the series, *Routines for Extraordinary Living* on Amazon and everywhere books are sold.

TOOLS FOR EXTRAORDINARY LIVING:

THE SNOOZE BUTTON SESSIONS

The secret of getting ahead is getting started.
The secret of getting started is
breaking your complex,
overwhelming tasks into small,
manageable tasks,
and then starting on the first one.

~ MARK TWAIN

A MESSAGE FROM KERRY: HOW THE SNOOZE BUTTON TRANSFORMED MY LIFE

If you come to a fork in the road, take it.

~YOGI BERRA

Let me take you back to a moment that changed my life… I was in Israel hiking with my family. We came to a beautiful clearing. There were trees arranged in a perfect circle around a giant space covered in pine needles. Birds were chirping, the sun was filtering down. Sounds were muffled. A sense of mystery hovered in the air. I sat down in the middle of the clearing, gazing at the trees around me. There was a feeling of expectancy in the air. I felt like I had been there before. The sense of *déjà vu* was strong.

Suddenly, I had a vivid flashback and I was transported back in time. It was as if I were watching a movie. I could see everything in perfect detail. In my mind's eye, I could see the younger Kerry, the younger me, sitting in the middle of a clearing just like the one I was in. There she was, alone in the woods, writing furiously in her journal. I had flashed back to a scene from my early 20s when I was living on a kibbutz in Israel. Those were tumultuous years for me, because I had dropped out of college in my senior year to travel the world. Upon reflection, it was not the best planning, I know, but back then, it seemed like a fantastic idea, a perfect plan—drop out of school and then drop out of life to become a world traveler. Nobody ever said young adults have great reasoning skills and I, for one, certainly didn't!

The younger version of me had gone to Israel to find myself by purposely losing myself. I had given away everything I owned except for my series of Hermann Hesse books and I hit the road with a backpack, $500 and a thirst for adventure. I was planning to completely drop out, no contact with anyone or anything for the entire year. No credit cards, no cellphone; it was just me and the world. Ok and a nice pair of heels. Perfect adventure travel attire, right? I wanted to *live* my life fully; I wanted to explore the world. I was always searching back then—searching, searching, ever searching—looking for the meaning of life.

I've always been a dreamer and a deep thinker. From my earliest memories, I questioned why some people have so much while others have so little. It seemed to me there were enough resources, they just weren't distributed properly. I never quite understood why we couldn't all "just get along." I was positive the world would be a better place if everyone just learned to share. Communal living was exactly what I envisioned. It was a dream come true for someone like me. Working together, eating together, living together—isn't this the way life was supposed to be? It certainly seemed that way for me. So when I learned that a kibbutz was an experiment in communal living, I had to try it. Off to Israel I went and onto the kibbutz I moved.

On the kibbutz, we worked and took classes in exchange for room, board and travel throughout Israel. Whenever I wasn't working on the kibbutz, I would spend time in nature. I loved to hike to a clearing right outside the kibbutz and ponder the great mysteries of the universe. I would sit and write in my journal, detailing all my hopes and dreams. This is exactly what I was doing on that day so many years before. I was sitting, writing in my journal and imagining what my perfect future would look like.

As I sat there 30 years later, I was swept away by the vividness of the memory. I flashed back to what I had written that day: Get married to a smart, kind man, have lots of kids, a big house with enough land for animals and a garden. Become an expert chef. There would be dinner on the table every single night and we would eat as a family. I would have a job I loved. The current me could see it all so clearly; it was like my younger self was sitting next to me and I was reading the journal as she wrote it. Those things I was writing long ago seemed so out of reach to the 22-year-old version of me. I wasn't sure how I could go from the young woman I was to the woman I wanted to become.

Yet, here I was, many years later, all grown up and I realized in a flash that all my dreams had come true. I was looking at my husband and my five kids. I was traveling with the very family I had once yearned to have. I had a job I loved. Everything I had written in that journal so many years prior had come true. Talk about a surreal, out of body moment; it was like the adult Kerry was standing behind the young Kerry, reading her journal and saying, "Check, check, check." In a flash, I realized that although I had acquired everything I had dreamed of all those years earlier, I still felt a deep yearning inside. How could this be, I wondered? Why was I so unfulfilled? If every single dream I had once dreamed had come to pass, why was I still feeling like something was missing? Why wasn't I happy? I sat in that clearing pondering how mysterious life truly is. I wondered, truly wondered, what was missing?

Then, it hit me. I knew what I had to do… I had to start dreaming again! That was the only way to recreate my life anew, to become the next grandest version of who I wanted to be. I needed to make a new list, dream new dreams—become a new me.

As soon as we made it back to the hotel, I sat down and wrote furiously. I began writing down anything and everything I dreamed of. I didn't hold back. I dreamed the most daring, glorious life I could imagine, no holds barred. I allowed myself to write down anything and everything that popped into my head. I was writing so fast; I didn't even know what I was writing.

When I was done, I sat back, satisfied and looked at what I had written: Spend more time with my kids and husband; spend more time outdoors; expand my career; write the book I always wanted to write; help more people; become an international speaker; enjoy more adventures; buy a beach house. It went on and on and on. As I stared at the list, I started to think the entire thing was silly. How was I going to do this? The doubts poured in.

I sat there, staring at my new dream-list and the doubts continued. Then I heard a voice. (No, I wasn't going crazy; it was my own voice.) The voice was from deep down inside me. The voice I never really listened to much because I was so busy doing the right thing, being responsible and adulting like crazy.

The voice said, "You can do anything you put your mind to. Once you decide, you will figure out how to make it work. Look at all you have accomplished until now. Just make the commitment and move forward." I made the decision in that moment to commit to accomplishing everything I dreamed of. I would create an epic life—the life of my dreams!

A few months after I had made my dream list, I made an effort to create some changes. But it was *hard*. I was resisting. My life was *busy*! I had no time for dream fulfillment. Most days I was just trying to get by—working, cooking, cleaning, chauffeuring my children around, sports, activities, laundry, pets… I had a lot of excuses. Then, something happened that truly changed my life.

One morning, the alarm clock sounded. I went to hit the snooze button, as usual. Something stopped me, a thought. Robin Sharma's thought, "To get the results that only 5% of the people get, you have to be willing to do what only 5% of the people are willing to do." I decided to hit the snooze but instead of going back to sleep, I meditated. When the alarm clock rang again, I turned it off, got up and started my day. I didn't think too much about it, I didn't know my entire *life* had just changed. But it had!

That day went really smoothly; it was so easy. I was calm, collected, relaxed all day long. Nothing could get to me. Not the guy cutting me off on the road, not the person who took my spot in the parking lot, not the student who didn't like my class, not my kids acting like kids do. I was unperturbed. No matter what happened, I was completely centered. I thought to myself, "What's different? Why is everything so easy today?" Then I remembered that I had meditated in the morning. Was that it?

I told my husband about this snooze technique and he tried using it. After trying it out for just one day, my husband told me it had been one of the best days of his life. This was interesting considering he had worked a full ten-hour day and then came home to the pandemonium that was our house. My husband grew quiet. We sat there, staring at each other, thrilled that we had found something so simple that could change the quality of our entire day. We agreed that we would continue doing this each day and maybe stretch or do yoga too. And that is what we did. Each day we would awaken and do our practices. And it was a true game changer.

I started to feel really, really *good!* I felt accomplished. Each day, before I even started my day, I had wins, serious wins. The simple act of getting up instead of snoozing helped me to create a healthy morning routine. This calm start to my day stood in marked contrast to waiting until the last moment to leap out of bed, trying to catch up with the day.

My life was changing, my body was changing and my mind was changing. I was centered. I was happy. My entire life was moving in an entirely different direction than ever before. Life became easy. And when life becomes easy, it frees up a lot of time to craft the life of dreams. So, that is exactly what I did.

At this same time, I began journaling daily. During one of my morning journaling sessions, I remembered that when I was a young girl, my greatest wish was to become a writer. I used to write poetry in my room when I was little. I knew I would be a writer one day. I didn't *think* it, I *knew* it. That was my life's path. As a young girl, I wrote all the time, but I never showed anyone my writing. Life had other plans for me, but it wasn't too late I decided. It's never too late.

The next day, during my morning snooze session, I started writing. It felt good; it felt right. I never planned to write an entire book and by no means was I planning on getting my book published. Writing was just for me. One day, I wrote the outline for this book and I began to think that this technique that I had accidentally stumbled upon had the capacity to create real, measurable change in people's lives. It was a simple way to do small, daily acts of greatness, which would then create new habits. It was a simple method to create new ways of thinking that would give the space for people to contemplate things they want to change in their lives.

I didn't just write about a method to create real, positive change, I lived it. The more I incorporated these morning practices into my life, the better my life got. My conviction grew that this could help other people. I started to teach these ideas to my students and then, one day, I taught an entire class on using the snooze button to meditate, journal, exercise or read. I was teaching my theories. It was happening! And the best part was that people were telling me that it was changing their lives. They were finally meditating or exercising or journaling. It worked for them just as it had worked for me! And it was easy.

As I taught the snooze button ideas, they became a lot more real to me, everything became clear. I asked for feedback from my students, I asked them to keep me up to date on their progress. I began using this material everywhere I worked. I incorporated the ideas into my work with corporate clients, teaching them stress reduction. I used the snooze button technique when I was teaching kids mindfulness. It was even applicable when I taught peak performance to athletic teams.

Life became magical. I became a better teacher and my students were getting better results. I was in flow. The most amazing part of it all was that these concepts were helpful to EVERYONE! As my business expanded, so did my belief that these ideas could help people transform their lives. The ideas evolved and this book is the result of that evolution.

What you have in your hands is a blueprint for creating and maintaining positive change in your life. This book is about taking action. This book is about getting results. It's a no-nonsense, no bullshit guide to creating change and transformation. The entire book is based on the idea that "big change starts small." We can create lasting, effective change in our lives by simply changing small things day by day.

It is said that "The journey of a thousand miles begins with one step." It is my wish that this book be that first step for you.

You can always begin again.
~ **SHARON SALZBURG**

XO Kerry

RESOURCES

Be Extraordinary Publishing, Inc.
Beextraordinarypublishing.com
Email: beextraordinarypublishing@gmail.com
Instagram: https://www.instagram.com/beextraordinarypublishing/

Kerry:
Kerryfishercoaching.com
Email: iamkerryfisher@gmail.com
LinkedIn: www.linkedin.com/in/kerry-fisher-
Instagram: https://www.instargram.com/iamkerryfisher/

Lawrence:
Email: lawrencetuazon84@gmail.com
Linkedin: https://www.linkedin.com/in/lawrence-tuazon-b32725239/
Instagram: https://www.instagram.com/lawrenceins/

LOOK FOR OTHER BOOKS FROM BE EXTRAORDINARY PUBLISHING, INC.

THE EXTRAORDINARY LIVING SERIES

The Extraordinary Living Series is a series of books with one central premise: You can live the life of your dreams, you can become the person you
dream of becoming. All it takes is action. The series teaches you the tools,
techniques and tips that will help you take control of your life, so that you
can create the masterpiece life you have always imagined.

TOOLS FOR EXTRAORDINARY LIVING: THE SNOOZE BUTTON SESSIONS BY KERRY B. FISHER

Book 1 in the Extraordinary Living Series

Tools for Extraordinary Living: The Snooze Button Sessions is the first book in
the Extraordinary Living Series. This is the book that started it all. The Snooze
Button Technique was born out of an epiphany Kerry Fisher had one day while
hiking with her family. She came into a clearing in the woods and suddenly
flashed back to a scene from her youth where she had been in a similar clearing, writing down all her hopes and dreams for her future. As the adult Kerry
remembered what the young Kerry had written, she realized all her dreams
had come true. Which was great. Except for one thing: she still wasn't happy.

This revelation set Kerry on a journey of personal growth and transformation which completely changed her life, her family's life and the
direction of her career. You see, Kerry had discovered that we all know
what we have to do to have an incredible life, we just don't know how
to do it. So Kerry created the Snooze Button Technique to give people a
way to take action immediately. She began to share this technique with

her family, her students, her family and the results were incredible. Soon enough, people were reporting that they were changing, their life was changing. The results were so incredible that Kerry knew she had to share this technique with the world so she wrote this book to do just that. If you are ready to create change in your life, get the book today. It is filled with simple, nourishing practices that will supercharge your life.

ROUTINES FOR EXTRAORDINARY LIVING
BY KERRY B. FISHER

Book 2 in The Extraordinary Living Series

The second book in the extraordinary living series, *Routines for Extraordinary Living* is for those people who want to create change in their life but don't know where to start. The book takes you step by step through your day, teaching you how to establish nourishing routines throughout the day to move you towards the extraordinary life you deserve. This book is all about creating a lifestyle where healthy routines are woven into your day. You will create practices that are built into your everyday life that nourish your body, your mind and your spirit. Before you know it, your life will be one of ease and flow, which enables you to have the energy you need to create the life you desire.

MINDSET MASTERY FOR EXTRAORDINARY LIVING
BY KERRY B. FISHER

Book 3 in The Extraordinary Living Series

The third book in the extraordinary living series, *Mindset Mastery for Extraordinary Living* is for people who are ready to take their lives to the next level. The book goes deep into the science behind why we do what we do. You will learn about the way your brain and your nervous system work and how you can use your biology to create the life you have dreamed of. You will learn how to make goals that align with your true purpose here on earth and then you will create the plan to make those goals a reality. This book examines the way our emotions work, how our nervous system and brain seek to protect us and gives you the tools you need to rewire your brain so that you can create the masterpiece of a life that you deserve.

OTHER BOOKS TO LOOK FOR

TOTAL LIFE TRANSFORMATION
BY KERRY FISHER, LAWRENCE TUAZON

This book is a compilation of the amazing stories of transformation, written by everyday people who turned their ordinary lives into extraordinary lives. These are the stories of people who were tested to their very limits. People who experienced one of those dark moments of the soul when they realized they needed to totally transform their lives. Join us and learn about the way that these incredible people went from their lowest low to their very best life.

This book will inspire and uplift you. The stories will help you to realize that it is never too late to turn your life around. After all, we are all on a hero's journey. It is up to us to decide how we want that journey to go. Read this book. It will change your life.

THE QUEST FOR EXTRAORDINARY LIVING:
INSIGHTS ON THE JOURNEY TO EXTRAORDINARY
BY KERRY B. FISHER

During the global pandemic, Kerry decided to write an article every single day for a year. She began the project and it became a joyous practice. Each day Kerry would wait for inspiration to strike and would write the insight on a platform called Insights by Mindvalley. This series contains the insights Kerry wrote during that year.

One of Kerry's deepest wishes from a very young age was to be a writer. It was a secret dream she rarely shared with anyone.

On January 2, 2022, Kerry was sitting in her backyard reading The Alchemist by Paulo Coelho. The book is about a shepherd boy who was on a quest to find his life's purpose. As Kerry read the book, she asked herself one simple question, "What is my life's purpose?" She was surprised when the thought immediately jumped into her head, "You are here to write."

The next thought was this, "What does a writer do?"

The answer again jumped into her head, "A writer writes."

And as the sun rose over the horizon, on the second day of 2022, Kerry made a decision that she would write every day for an entire year. She decided to write on a platform called Insights by Mindvalley and each day for a full year, she wrote an insight. She didn't miss a day. The daily writing fueled her passion for writing. She decided to write a book on the tools she had discovered that helped her lead a great life and the Extraordinary Living series came to life.

One day, a friend told Kerry how much she had been enjoying Kerry's daily insights. She suggested that she publish them as an anthology. Over the next week, three other people said the same thing to her. And so, Kerry began the process of reading through her year of daily insights. She envisioned a new series, based on these simple stories of self reflection and deep soul searching.

The Insights series is a powerful reminder that every single person we meet is our teacher and every single event in our life can serve as a lesson. They remind you that you can become the person you dream of becoming, you can live the extraordinary life you imagine. It just takes an inquisitive mind and an open heart.

Check out all the books in the series and see what insights they bring for you.

MEDITATION FOR EXTRAORDINARY LIVING
BY KERRY B. FISHER

Meditation has long been used by many religious and spiritual traditions to tap into altered states of mind. The mystics from the ages used meditation to help them to move into deep states of awareness and consciousness. They found that meditation kept them calm in body, mind and spirit.

Meditation has become increasingly common across the world because it is one of the best ways to change your state of being. This book will teach you many different meditation techniques, so you can bring this practice into your life.

BREATHWORK FOR EXTRAORDINARY LIVING
BY KERRY B. FISHER

Breathwork is one of the easiest ways to change your mental, emotional and physical state. Breath practices have been used throughout time to help people to stay calm, cool and collected. They have also been used to achieve higher states of consciousness. This book is a book intended to give you some of the science behind breathing practices, as well as providing a multitude of amazing practices to bring into your life. Check it out if you want to add this amazing practice into your life.

BE EXTRAORDINARY PUBLISHING

Our mission is to show you how to be the very best version of yourself, how to live the very best life you can possibly live. Our books are all about bringing attention to all the important areas of your life, so that you can uplevel them all.

We also provide a wide array of services for authors and aspiring authors looking to create their own masterpiece.

Please check our website at beextraordinarypublishing.com for more details.

We publish books on a variety of health and wellness topics, as well as on peak performance and mindset. We focus on personal transformation and teach you how you can live your best life. Look for books on a wide variety of topics including nutrition, exercise, yoga, pilates, meditation, breathwork, mindfulness practices and self care.

Our books will show you how you can upgrade your life using simple techniques, tips and tricks to create a magnificent life.

We also bring you stories of the heroes amongst us. Stories of the journey towards extraordinary living. These books illuminate how every person is on a Hero's Journey, how every person is on a journey towards the extraordinary. Look for our books on Amazon, in bookstores and everywhere books are sold.

ABOUT THE AUTHORS

LAWRENCE TUAZON

Lawrence Tuazon is a health and fitness coach, a speaker and a peak performance expert. He is an amputee who has inspired thousands of people around the world with his radical health transformation.

As the founder of Total Health Coaching, Lawrence guides his clients on their journey towards peak health and fitness. Lawrence is passionate about helping his clients achieve permanent health and body transformation by encouraging them to take a holistic approach to achieve extraordinary health. His clients get results due to Lawerence's dedication to creating a tailored plan that works for them.

Lawrence is passionate about all aspects of wellness including nutrition, exercise and mindset. His vision is to create chronic health as the new normal instead of chronic disease and to bring holistic health education into the school curriculum. Lawrence believes that everybody can lead a life of extraordinary health and wellness and he has dedicated his life to this pursuit.

Contact Info:
Email: lawrencetuazon84@gmail.com
Linkedin: https://www.linkedin.com/in/lawrence-tuazon-b32725239/
Instagram: https://www.instagram.com/lawrenceins/

KERRY FISHER

Kerry was raising a family and working as an attorney when she began a daily yoga practice. She immediately noticed that yoga was the perfect antidote to her hectic lifestyle. Initially interested in yoga as a physical practice that made her feel good in her body, Kerry soon realized yoga was a lot more than that. She decided to take a teacher training and immediately began teaching. Kerry eventually left her law career and began to focus on teaching and coaching full time.

Kerry's mission is to help others find a more balanced and fulfilled life. She believes in action and has created a system that is easy to implement so that people can create change quickly. Kerry teaches Simple Tips for Extraordinary Living using stress reduction techniques and work-life balance to help people supercharge their lives. She coaches corporate clients and elite athletes in mindset and peak performance techniques and creates tailored programs for private clients who are seeking mastery in all areas of their lives.

After many years of teaching and coaching, Kerry is focused on writing, creating courses and speaking on the topics she is so passionate about. She is on a mission to inspire and encourage people to become the person they dream of being and to create the life they imagine.

When not teaching or writing, you can usually find Kerry somewhere outdoors with her five children in tow.

FOR FURTHER INFORMATION

Thank you for reading this book. It is our hope that you received a lot of value from the material presented here. It is also our desire that this book will help you become the next greatest and healthiest version of yourself.

This is the first in a series of co-authored books on Health and Holistic Living. Each book contains the stories of coaches, elite athletes, wellness educators and everyday people as they share the secrets they have discovered for living their healthiest life.

We aim to find authors who have simple tips that are easy to put into action. We believe that action is the only way to live the healthiest life. We all know what to do, the books in this series tell you how to do it.

If you enjoyed this book, please leave a review on the site where you purchased it.

Please share this book with anyone who you think could benefit from the information in this book.